SO-ACI-496

Feeling Great

&

Looking Good...

A CHRISTIAN'S GUIDE
TO WOMEN'S HEALTH
AND WEIGHT CONTROL

...FOR THE CAUSE OF CHRIST

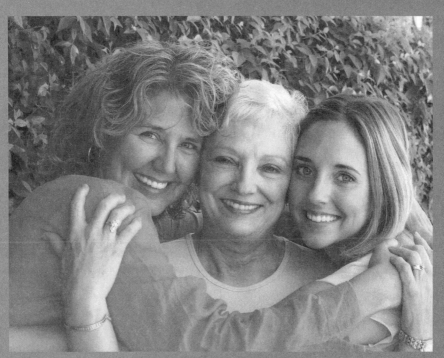

JANE GRAFTON

Copyright © 2006
CHRISTIAN WOMANHOOD
8400 Burr Street
Crown Point, Indiana 46307

www.christianwomanhood.org

ISBN: 0-9745195-8-8

All Scriptures in this book are taken from the 1611 King James Bible.

CREDITS:
Cover Design: Gina Eyer
Manuscript Design: Linda Stubblefield
Art: Karyn Hermann

OTHER BOOKS BY JANE GRAFTON
Marlene Evans: A Biography
Losing Weight ~ Gaining Control
True Stories for Moms
True Stories for Wives Only

Disclaimer: Using a quote by a certain writer does not mean the author is giving blanket endoresement on that person's works. The quoted matter has been reprinted exactly as it appeared in the source material.

Printed in the United States of America

Dedication

I lovingly dedicate this book to the women who are struggling with their health and with weight control. I love you; I have prayed for you; and I admire you for seeking answers. I have no doubt that God has great things for you to accomplish in your lifetime. I pray this book will give you the answers you are needing to regain your health and the wisdom to be more effective for Him so that you will make a tremendous impact for eternity!

Jane Grafton

About the Author

Jane Grafton is the wife of Tom Grafton and the mother of one daughter, Carissa. The Graftons are active members of First Baptist Church of Hammond, Indiana, where Jane serves with Tom in the Truck Stop Chapel Ministry. She also teaches the Friendship Class, an adult ladies' Sunday school class.

After graduating from Bible college in 1972, Jane taught fourth grade at First Baptist Schools in Rosemount, Minnesota, for several years. In 1977 she moved to Indiana to attend Hyles-Anderson College.

Jane was employed by Hyles-Anderson College from 1978 until 1986, at which time she began working for Christian Womanhood, a ministry of First Baptist Church of Hammond, Indiana, under the leadership of Marlene Evans. She is now the Managing Editor for Christian Womanhood under the leadership of Dr. and Mrs. Jack Schaap. Jane is also a conference speaker and an author.

Acknowledgments

I want to thank my husband Tom and my daughter Carissa for the vital role they played in the publication of this book. Without my husband's patience and encouragement during my darkest days with my health, I would not be where I am today. He has been a Rock of Gibraltar to me. I respect him, I love him, and I am honored to be his wife. He is a wonderful, humble Christian who has been a tremendous husband. I also want to thank our daughter Carissa for her extra help at home, especially in the final days near my deadline! She is a great cook, cleaner, and organizer—all with a positive attitude. I am so pleased she has chosen to serve God with her life, to walk with Him daily, and to honor Him with her sweet Christian testimony.

I want to thank my pastor's wife, Mrs. Cindy Schaap, who is also my boss, my mentor, and my friend. I'm grateful for her belief in me and her encouragement through nearly five years of working together in Christian Womanhood. She has believed in me when I did not believe in myself. One of my favorite thoughts about Mrs. Schaap is that I know she prays for me on a regular basis.

I want to thank my preacher, Dr. Jack Schaap, pastor of First Baptist Church of Hammond, Indiana. He has paid a great price to be able to deliver wonderful truths of Scripture to his congregation at every church service. I am convinced that I would not be where I am today spiritually nor where I am with my health and weight control if it were not for the life-changing truths he has taught that I have been able to understand and institute into my daily life.

I want to thank Linda Stubblefield, my friend and co-worker, for doing the layout and graphic design of this book. It was a wonderful day when God allowed Linda to become a part of the Christian Womanhood staff. She is the senior member of our staff as Linda was hired to work for Christian Womanhood long before any of the rest of us. (That fact, however, does *not* make her the oldest member of our staff!) God has gifted Linda in the area of graphic arts and layout design. She is a master, and I'm thrilled she is on our team! I cannot find words to adequately express my gratitude for her patience with me under deadlines and for her willingness to care for so many details of this book.

I want to thank each of the Christian Womanhood office staff for "taking up the slack" while I was out of the office working on this project. This is a great group of ladies, and I count it a tremendous privilege to serve with them: Lisa Bates, Julie Busby, Rachael Christner, Colleen Clark, Michelle Cowling, Gina Eyer, Carissa Grafton, Joy Houghton, Sarah Martin, Kalynn Suba, Jeannie Mae Walker, Janice Wolfe, Rachel Wolfe, and Nanci Wonson. What a team who each have a servant's spirit and are of one mind to work together to accomplish the agenda of our senior editor, Mrs. Cindy Schaap. They are simply the best!

I want to thank Linda Flesher and Rena Fish for proofreading this manuscript. It is a great comfort to me to know that they will carefully read my writing and make the necessary corrections to make this a first-class publication.

I want to thank Carol Tudor, a registered nurse and my dear friend of 30 years, for reading this book as a medical professional. I was thrilled when she agreed to read it to help insure its accuracy regarding women's health.

I want to thank my sister, Joan Sullivan, a wonderful, soul-winning Christian for opening her lovely home to me when I needed some big chunks of time to be alone to finish the writing of this book. My thought is that "everyone needs a 'Joan' in her life." I am so thrilled God gave me one in my "baby" sister! I spent hours on the deck of her house typing on my laptop computer with hummingbirds "buzzing" past my head on their way to and from the feeder, hearing the chatter of beautiful black squirrels and chipmunks, listening to the song of the redbirds, and enjoying the tree-covered sand dune, flowers, and other plants in her backyard.

I want to thank Molly Audiss, my niece Theresa Carter, and her husband Daryl Carter for helping with some of the research of this book. I needed them and they came through for me!

I want to thank Karyn Hermann for her help with cartoon art work. She was introduced to me by her sister Chris Berger, a Hyles-Anderson College graduate, who was one of "my girls" when I was a dormitory supervisor.

Lastly, I want to thank my Lord and Saviour Jesus Christ for saving me and for directing my steps. He has been good to me in these 38 years since I received assurance of my salvation in May of 1968—just a few days before I graduated from high school. I had no idea what the future held for me, but how rewarding it has been to watch Him order my steps. God is good!

Table of Contents

Table of Contents

(continued)

Disclaimer

My mother was a nurse; her brother (my uncle) is a doctor; my sister Jan is a pediatric intensivist at Kosair Children's Hospital in Louisville, Kentucky; my younger sister Joan is a physician assistant to a prominent neurosurgeon in Michigan; I have two sisters-in-law and a close friend who are registered nurses; I have another very close friend who is a respiratory therapist; I have several cousins who are physicians and several who are nurses.

From my earliest memories I wanted to be a nurse and read every "Sue Barton" fiction book I could get my hands on. As a child I would look at my mother's memorabilia from nursing school and from the years she worked as a registered nurse before she married my dad, and I would dream of a nursing career. I have always had an interest in the medical field.

However, God's will did not lead me into the medical profession. I was greatly disappointed at the time, but looking back I see He was being good to me in not letting me pursue that path. He had other wonderful plans for my life.

As the author of this book on women's health, I fully realize that I am not a trained medical professional. Nor, in spite of all my relationships with professionally trained medical personnel, did their training rub off on me by the process of osmosis!

As you read, please keep in mind that this manuscript is not meant to be a textbook for medical professionals. Rather, it is written by a woman who has experienced a myriad of health issues in her lifetime, who for a number of years could not seem to get the help she needed, and who found much help through a wonderful Christian physician, long hours of research, and and some major lifestyle changes.

In no way am I trying to take the place of a trained medical professional to diagnose your problems or to treat your symptoms. I highly recommend that you find a principled holistic physician who will guide you and work with you in your pursuit of good health.

I have worked diligently to present accurate information. Much of what I have written I have learned by reading and researching information from trained medical professionals. I do ask for your mercy as you read this manuscript. You may read ideas with which you disagree. You have that right, but keep in mind that the principles I am teaching are principles which have helped me to regain my health.

It seems like a lifetime ago that I would go home and not know if I had the strength to climb to the top of the steps, walk into the bedroom, and fall into bed. Those are distant memories but memories that are responsible for the burden I have to help other women who are currently experiencing the same type of poor health that I once had or who seem to be headed in that direction.

Through some of the most difficult days, I wondered why God was allowing the struggles with my health. I believe one reason was so that I could eventually help other ladies. If just one person has her life transformed and is able to multiply her work for the Lord as a result, this book has been worth all of the time, effort, prayers, and love I have put into it. I am honored you have chosen to read it.

Whether you are suffering some major health issues or if you simply want to lose a few pounds and learn a healthier lifestyle in the process, I believe this book will be a help to you as you begin to establish the principles in your life.

Introduction

My quest for good health and proper weight control has been a long journey. It began a number of years ago and has been an evolution of sorts. I spent a number of years thinking I was destined to a life of fatigue, obesity, and physical ailments. It was a wonderful day when I realized that the state of my health is in my hands, and that I could do many things to help restore my health. (I am not discounting the vital role God plays; rather, I am emphasizing that the decisions and choices I make based on His principles determine my health—apart from a cataclysmic health issue He chooses for me.)

I have found that my story is not such an unusual one. I sometimes speak on the subject of women's health at ladies' conferences, and when I give my testimony, I always have a number of ladies say something like, "You could have used my name today when you were speaking. I felt like you were giving my testimony." They also tell me, "I wish I'd heard this 10 or 15 years ago!"

While there are numbers of women who identify with my story, there are also women who don't seem to relate at all to what I say. Perhaps they have lived a moderate lifestyle, especially in the area of food intake, and for whatever reasons, they have not had the extreme health problems I address. If you are one of those ladies, my prayer is that you will use this book to gain some understanding of women whom you may view as "hypochondriacs." I hope you will use this book as a tool to help those ladies. I know there are women who seem to enjoy being sick, who want to talk every detail of their sickness to everyone who will listen (numerous times!!!!), but don't seem to want answers. They seem content to remain in their state of poor health. However, I do not believe that is the majority.

I have two sisters who have not had the health issues I've experienced. I appreciate the fact that they have been very patient and understanding with me. Most of all, I appreciate their support through the years and the fact that they have not been judgmental of me. I know I have made some less-than-wise medical choices at times, but never have they expressed their disapproval of me. What great sisters I have! As sisters in Christ, it is my desire that we would treat each other in that same manner. Matthew 7:1 says, *"Judge not, that ye be not judged."* There's an old Indian proverb that says, "Don't criticize a man until you have walked two moons in his moccasins." It is far better to be understanding and kind to someone who may be undeserving of that treatment than to judge and criticize someone who genuinely has health issues. For those women who seem addicted to their poor health and the lifestyle that goes with it, they have an even greater need to be loved, accepted, and encouraged than those who are experiencing only physical maladies!

The more I have researched women's health and the more I have spoken on the subject, the more I realize there are vast numbers of women suffering with poor health. Sadly, I find that many of these ladies are suffering alone. Many have come to an almost victim mind set and feel there is nothing they can do; they believe their poor health and all of the aches, pains, and fatigue they are experiencing is just a part of growing old and something they have to accept and live with the rest of their lives.

My sister-in-law Kris Grafton (a registered nurse) and I visited a lady who, though only 60 years of age, is nearly an invalid. We walked into her nicely decorated home and were greeted in very dim surroundings. Because the light hurt her eyes, the shades were all closed and only one small light was on. She was shaky and dizzy. She feels old, overweight, and defeated. She believes

her life is over. *She's only 60!* That is young…and looking younger all the time as I approach my fifty-sixth birthday at this writing! (My birthday is November 13 just in case you want to send me a card!) I believe God has much for this dear lady to do in her lifetime, but she is nearly paralyzed in her lifestyle by poor health.

She asked Kris to take a look at her medications, one of which was an anti-depressant. She's been on it for four years and is no better. In fact, she is worse now than she was four years ago when she started taking it. This lady feels helpless, old, and useless. How sad! I believe there is much hope for this woman—and for every woman who is struggling with her health. The fact is, most of us simply do not have to suffer helplessly through old age.

One of the greatest attributes of God is that He is a God of principles and procedures. When we go haplessly through life, we find that life "happens" to us. We become victims of our circumstances, and negative things befall us. However, when we become principled in any area of our lives, we suddenly find that we are no longer victims. Applying right principles to our lives gives us success. We may not have success overnight, and we may have violated some principles which have caused some permanent damage. For example, if you are a diabetic who has had a toe—or a foot or a leg—removed because of gangrene, it is very unlikely (I think "impossible" would be the correct term) that it will grow back!

That just doesn't happen. But in whatever stage of health we find ourselves, applying right principles to our lifestyle will improve our health.

The principles I am presenting in this book are principles that have improved my health dramatically. They work. My prayer is that these principles will be practical, helpful, and easy for you to understand and put into practice. My prayer is that your health will be changed by applying the principles you read and that you will be able to do much more for eternity than you ever dreamed because of regained health.

On a lighter note, you will notice a number of one-liners, cartoons, and humorous anecdotes on many of the pages of this book. They have a purpose. I want to help you laugh. Laughter is healing. Proverbs 17:22a says, *"A merry heart doeth good like a medicine."* The issues in this book can become a little laborious and somewhat overwhelming. I'm wanting to help you live on the brighter side of life as you work to regain your health. Enjoy the humor and please don't take anything personally or let it offend you. Remember, the reason I placed them in this book is to help you enjoy life more!

I have prayed for you as I have prepared to write this book and as I have sat at the computer and typed the manuscript. I will continue to pray for you after this book is printed. God has put you in my heart, and I love you.

God bless you, dear reader!

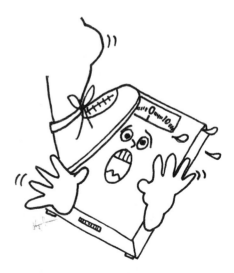

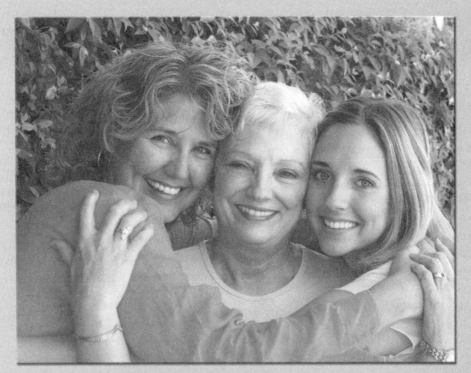

PART ONE

The Reality of Women's Health

My Story:
Dark Days and Sleepless Nights

I don't remember ever really feeling *great* as an adult…at least not for more than a few days or a few weeks at a time. I almost always felt tired; I had problems with my monthly cycle; I had numerous allergies, and I seemed to have constant sore throats from sinus drainage. It did not seem life should have to be that way, but no one ever seemed to be able to help me, even the medical community.

I now realize that many of my problems were due to my violating some very basic health principles—especially my eating habits. (I made some very poor choices that led to many of my problems. I can blame no one but myself for the years of bad health I endured.) But even with not feeling great, I could pretty much care for my priorities and my responsibilities.

However, about a year and a half after our daughter Carissa was born, I began struggling in a far greater way. My monthly cycle became more severe, and my energy levels dropped to a new low. I was also gaining weight that no diet seemed

to help. I went to the doctor and was told there was nothing wrong with me.

I continued having these symptoms over the next few years only to see them increase in intensity. Soon after I turned 40, I was diagnosed with endometriosis, and my gynecologist recommended a D&C. I had a brief respite from some of my symptoms but not for long, and he soon recommended a hysterectomy. I can recall facing that surgery with the attitude, "Finally, all of my hormone problems will be over. I will no longer have a monthly cycle, and I'm going to finally be able to get this excess weight off!" For some reason I had the impression that a hysterectomy would help me lose weight.

Boy, was I in for a shock! New health issues surfaced almost immediately. At my six-week checkup after surgery, my blood pressure was elevated. That was surprising to me as I had never experienced blood pressure issues. The nurse shook it off and said, "Probably your high reading is from being nervous. That happens to a lot of people when they are at a doctor's office."

However, a few months later I began having terrible headaches. As they increased both in frequency and intensity, I talked with my sister-in-law Kris who said, "Why don't we take your blood pressure?" It was 200 over 120 (normal is 120/70). She immediately scheduled an appointment for me to see the doctor, and I was put on blood pressure medication and bed rest until my blood pressure was down to a more normal rate. I was disappointed at having to take a second medication as my gynecologist had put me on Premarin (synthetic estrogen replacement therapy) after my hysterectomy.

Soon I was feeling very, very depressed. I woke up every morning with a dark cloud over me that stayed with me all day long. I was also continuing to gain weight. When I mentioned this to my gynecologist, he said, "You know, in order to lose weight you need to eat less!" I was humiliated and frustrated. ***I was eating less, but I was gaining more.*** (Later I would realize that I was breaking some basic principles of health such as skipping meals, not eating the right foods, etc.)

> Amazing! You hang something in your closet for a while, and it shrinks two sizes!

I talked with my general practitioner about my depression. He said it could be the blood pressure medication, so he switched me to another medication. My blood pressure had gone down from the original 200/120, but it was still elevated with a reading of about 150/95. I began the new medication, but the depression remained and so did my slightly elevated readings. I have since come to learn that nearly every—if not all—hypertension drug causes depression.

Life during these five-plus years after my hysterectomy is, in many ways, a blur to me. I went through each day feeling extremely fatigued most of the time. I then began having other health issues. Pain! I can't really explain the extreme pain to someone who has never experienced it, but some days my whole body hurt so badly that I couldn't stand for people to touch me. Other symptoms included cloudy thinking, forgetfulness, thinning hair (I mean thinning to the point I was going bald), dry hair, dry skin, insomnia, and general malaise.

My insomnia was severe. I just could not get to sleep at night. I would lie in bed awake until 2:00, 3:00, or 4:00 in the morning. Then when it was time to get up, of course, I was exhausted and could barely get out of bed. I had to get up because I had to take our daughter Carissa to school, but I experienced terrible fatigue all day long. The weight gain continued, and I felt like the Goodyear Blimp.

I was also an emotional wreck. I found myself irritable and snappy at situations that normally would never have bothered me. I would get frustrated at our grade-school-age daughter over the smallest things. I recall pounding on the kitchen counter and yelling at her one morning as we were about to leave for school. When I realized what I was doing, I stopped and thought, "Who (or what!) has invaded my body?!" I was like a crazy woman. I apologized to her and she, of course, sweetly forgave me.

Then she said, "I'm sorry, Mom, but I still don't understand what you were upset about."

The sad thing was I didn't know either! I worked hard not to allow such out-of-control actions to happen again, but feelings of frustration were common for me, and I know I sometimes had an edge in my voice that she did not deserve.

My health seemed to go from bad to worse, and about a year and a half after my hysterectomy, I felt the worst I had felt in my life. I had many of the symptoms listed below. Maybe you'll recognize a number of them from your own personal experiences.

- Arthritis
- Autoimmune diseases such as lupus, fibromyalgia, and rheumatoid arthritis
- Bad breath
- Breast cancer
- Cravings (for the wrong types of food, of course!)
- Depression
- Dry, scaly scalp
- Dry skin
- Extreme fatigue
- Extremely painful periods
- Fat gain, especially around the abdomen, hips, and thighs
- Fibroid tumors
- Fibrocystic breasts
- Foggy thinking
- Gall bladder disease
- Hereafter syndrome (walking into a room and can't remember what you're "here after!")
- Insomnia (can't get to sleep at night and can't wake up in the morning)
- Irregular periods
- Irritability
- Low libido
- Obesity
- Osteoporosis
- Pain
- PMS
- Thinning hair (including pubic and underarm hair)

> Scales are for fish— not women!

Though I did not experience every single symptom listed above, I did have a majority of them. It was a very depressing thought that I would have to live the rest of my life in such poor health.

Eventually I got to a point where I felt like the side effects of my medications exceeded any benefit I might be receiving, so I quit taking them. That did help my depression somewhat, but I still struggled tremendously because of my poor health. I am grateful that I never went on any type of anti-depressant drugs! God protected me.

My future seemed very bleak. Though I never contemplated suicide there were a number of days I wished for God to take me home to Heaven. I longed for the pain, the depression, the fatigue, and all of the other symptoms to just go away!

I also felt very alone at this time because I'd been told that nothing was wrong with me. Though I did not believe I was being a hypochondriac, I felt that others would think of me as such since I had not been given a diagnosis; I just had a long list of symptoms. At one point I was diagnosed with fibromyalgia. I received warnings by several medical professionals not to use that term as it is frowned upon by the medical community who view it more as a catch-all "diagnosis" for women who have a lot of complaints rather than a real disease. One of the most frustrating recommendations I received was to see a psychiatrist. I knew in that physician's mind I was mentally, not physically ill.

Though these were very dark days for me, I have no doubt that God allowed all of this for a purpose. I believe He wanted to do a work in my life. I do not believe I suffered near what many others have suffered with their health. I never had to endure chemotherapy, radiation, Alzheimer's, or many other difficulties that are much worse than what I experienced. I am grateful to God for allowing these trying times. I wish I could say I always had a grateful attitude to God for what I was experiencing. I did not. But I do believe that as I learned some lessons that God had for me (one of which was to be a praising and grateful Christian no matter what the circumstances), God began to bring me out of the wilderness where I was living.

God was gracious to me in many ways. One of the greatest was in giving me such a godly, patient husband, Tom Grafton, who was so understanding through these difficult times. Never did I sense a critical or judgmental tone in his voice or in his actions. He helped tremendously with our young daughter, and he helped me with the housework or whatever else I seemed to need. I admire him, I love him, and I am indebted to him beyond words!

> Husband to wife:
> A headache that lasts for 17 months is a problem. See a doctor.

Help Was on the Way

My poor health was seriously affecting every area of my life—spiritually, emotionally, and physically. It limited my church attendance as I often did not seem to have the strength to go to evening services; I was not nearly as effective as I had been in my soul winning; my prayer life was affected—though I did keep reading my Bible and praying daily. I had been to several doctors including a major medical center and had been told repeatedly that nothing was wrong with me. I knew that if there was any hope for my health situation, it was through God. He was my only hope. I prayed and prayed. I poured out my heart to God and begged for answers. He heard my prayers.

He used a dear, close friend, Carol Tudor, to help me take the first step in regaining my health. One day she said, "Jane, why don't you make an appointment with Dr. Cal Streeter to see if he can help you." (Dr. Streeter is a holisitic physician who is a member of our church. He is now retired and is on staff at First Baptist Church of Hammond, Indiana, as a medical consultant.) I did not realize it at the time, but one of Dr.

Streeter's strongest areas as a physician is women's health.

I was hesitant to make that appointment as I felt I would just pay more money to hear that nothing was wrong with me. However, I discussed it with my husband, and he encouraged me to see Dr. Streeter as soon as possible. I did make that appointment, and it was a turning point for my health.

The first thing I noticed was that Dr. Streeter listened to me. He asked questions, let me answer those questions, made notes while I was answering, and then asked more questions. He did not have a few pat answers to pacify me. He listened, and then he said, "We're going to find the problem and get you well!" That in itself gave me hope. He took me seriously, and he believed me.

Dr. Streeter ordered blood work and had me schedule another appointment. On that second visit, he went over my blood work and explained each test result. He made two changes that gave me immediate help and that gave me hope for the future. First, he discovered that I had a hypothyroid condition, so he prescribed some much-needed thyroid medication. The second step was putting me on bioidentical hormone replacement therapy of natural progesterone. Within two weeks I had taken a very small, but very noticeable, step forward. For the first time in several years, I was able to go to sleep much better at night, I woke up feeling somewhat rested in the morning, my energy levels were up, and I was more able to function each day. Eventually I even began, ever so slowly, taking off some of the weight I had packed on during my years of terribly ill health.

Though I was not immediately healed of all my nagging symptoms, that first step began my journey of taking my health into my own hands. I began to realize that my health is *my* responsibility. I also realized it meant I was going to have to do research—not only in the medical realm, but also in the Scriptural realm. I needed to institute a Biblically based program into my life in order to have the best health possible. I had a lot to learn,

especially about what it means to eat a healthy, balanced diet; to get enough sleep; and to have balanced hormones.

That appointment with Dr. Streeter was about ten years ago. Sometimes regaining my health has been a real struggle, both physically and spiritually. There are times I have taken some steps backward, but God has been very gracious. For example, after several years on the thyroid medication, it seemed to quit working. Through trial and error with several different medications, Dr. Streeter discovered the medication (Thyrolar) that works best for me—which even helped control some health issues that the original medication did not, such as lowering my blood pressure.

Though I am still doing some "fine tuning" to try to get my body into balance, I've come a long way from the person who didn't think she could make it up the steps to her bedroom when she got home. I believe my journey has been longer than it will be for many who read this book as my journey was somewhat "trial and error." Many times I did not realize the importance of some of the things I did or did not do. It has been a learning process for me, and sometimes a "re-learning" process!

As I look back, I realize that if I had been more proactive in my approach and begun the research much earlier I would probably not have gotten into such an extreme situation.

There were two hindrances to my doing that.

1. I just trusted what the doctors said.

A woman was not feeling well, so she visited her doctor. The good doctor, after giving her a thorough examination, said grimly, "Mrs. Goode, I am sorry to have to say this, but if you want to get well again you will have to lose a foot."

"What!?! You mean my foot has to be amputated?"

"Oh, no, no..." replied the good doctor, "I mean you have to lose a foot from around your waistline!"

When they told me there was nothing wrong, I believed them and felt I was just being a wimp about my symptoms.

2. The worse my health became, the less energy I had to even think of finding answers. My mind was so foggy I did not seem to be able to think in solutions. That's why it was so important that I listened to my husband and to others who loved me (like Carol Tudor) as they had a much better perspective than I had. Because I had so little energy and my mind was foggy, I was lulled into thinking there were no solutions. I am so glad I had several people who were willing to take on the fight for me when I was too weak to do so. I am also grateful God gave me the character and the wisdom to try to do what these people said.

Money talks; chocolate sings!

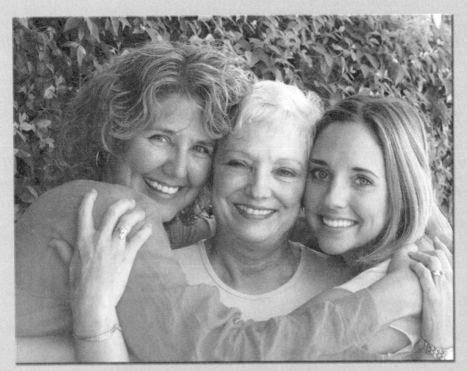

PART TWO

God's Will Regarding Women's Health

"That Thou Mayest...Be in Health..."

III John verse 2 states, *"Beloved, I wish above all things that thou mayest prosper and be in health, even as thy soul prospereth."* The apostle John was saying, "I don't just want you to prosper spiritually; I also want you to prosper physically and to be in good health."

The word *health* occurs 17 times in the Bible, and the word *healing* is used 14 times. Of course, the big purpose of Jesus' miracles was to win the lost to Himself so they would have eternal life, but the majority of His miracles involved healing the sick. Matthew 4:23 says, *"And Jesus went about all Galilee, teaching in their synagogues, and preaching the gospel of the kingdom, and healing all manner of sickness and all manner of disease among the people."* Jesus' heartbeat was always winning the lost, but He was also very interested in bringing good health to people while He walked on this earth.

Hebrews 13:8 says, *"Jesus Christ the same yesterday, and to day, and for ever."* If, while Jesus lived on this earth, He was interested in the health of the people whom He had created, He is just as interested today. While I believe that God sometimes chooses people for the "furnace of affliction" to try them or to use them in an unusual way, I also believe the Bible teaches that it is His will for most people to have good health most of the time.

It seems that Marlene Evans, the founder of Christian Womanhood, was one of those people God chose for the furnace of affliction. Through nearly 20 years of fighting breast cancer and then ovarian cancer, stage IV, she was a rejoicing Christian. Her ministry to Christian ladies seemed to flourish as she struggled through chemotherapy treatments, surgeries, and all the side effects of the medications and surgeries. I admired that lady in a great way as I worked "up close" with her and saw that what she taught publicly was what she lived privately. She was a wonderful Christian lady who had a very close walk with God. It seemed God gave her miraculous grace to live "above the clouds" even through her darkest days with cancer until she went to Heaven on July 8, 2001.

Marlene Evans was a

Despite the cost of living, have you noticed how it remains so popular?

remarkable Christian, one of my heroes, and a woman whose life I try to emulate. I am admitting my weakness as a Christian, and I wish it were not so, but the fact is, I am not a very good Christian—I am no "Marlene Evans" when I am sick! Sickness affects my Bible reading and prayer, my church attendance, my attitudes and my spirit, and my life in every other area. I am not saying that people who are sick are not right with God, nor am I saying that sickness is an excuse not to obey the principles of the Word of God. What I am saying is that it seems I am able to accomplish much more for eternity when I have energy, a clear mind, and good health than when I am not well.

Dr. Jack Hyles was the pastor of First Baptist Church of Hammond, Indiana, for over 40 years. He was my pastor for almost 24 of those years.

Second Opinion

A woman had not been feeling well and went to the doctor for a checkup. After the physical examination and a battery of blood tests and x-rays, she asked the doctor about her situation.

The doctor replied, "You are very sick. You might not live longer than perhaps three or four months."

The woman, in despair, yet with a glimpse of hope said, "If you don't mind, Doctor, I'd like to have a second opinion."

"Okay," the doctor replied, "You're ugly too!"

On Sunday, December 17, 1995, he preached a sermon from I Thessalonians 5:23 which says, *"And the very God of peace sanctify you wholly; and I pray God your whole spirit and soul and body be preserved blameless unto the coming of our Lord Jesus Christ."* I wrote the following notes in my Bible from that sermon: "The soul dwells in the body, and the spirit dwells in the soul. Therefore, I must keep my body healthy to keep my soul healthy to keep my spirit healthy for the Holy Spirit to dwell in." He also used III John 1, 2 as another Scripture reference, *"The elder unto the wellbeloved Gaius, whom I love in the truth. Beloved, I wish above all things that thou mayest prosper and be in health, even as thy soul prospereth."*

One of Dr. Hyles' foremost teachings was that, in order to be effective Christians, we are to live the Holy Spirit-filled life. He understood and taught the importance of taking good care of the temple (the body) God has given us so that we might be more effective in our work for Him. He never taught, nor am I teaching, that it is impossible to be filled with the Holy Spirit if we are sick. However, most of us are able to accomplish much more for eternity as we live a disciplined, Spirit-filled life where we take the necessary steps to keep our bodies healthy. Dr. Hyles taught a Wednesday night Bible study series on the Holy Spirit and then had those lessons compiled into a book *Meet the Holy Spirit*. Reading and studying that book would give you great insight on the Spirit-filled life and would help you in the matter of caring for your body, especially the chapter entitled, "A Spirit-Controlled, Mind-Controlled Body."

When a person trusts Christ as Saviour, there is one main reason that God leaves him on this earth. We are made to praise Him and should do so while we are on this earth, but we can praise Him in Heaven. We are to grow spiritually and should do so while we are on this earth, but we can learn and grow in Heaven. There is one thing we are to do that we can do only on this earth, and that is to influence others spiritually. More specifically, we are here to win others to Christ and to teach them to do the same. More often than not, most of us are more effective doing the work God has for us when we are in good health.

The pursuit of good health is a very Scriptural and spiritual pursuit if we are doing so in order to increase our work and effectiveness for eternity.

My friend and co-worker, Loretta Walker, began having struggles with her health in her early forties. She has written the following paragraphs that I believe will be helpful to you. She has graciously allowed me to include these thoughts in this book:

"In August of the year I turned 40, my body changed drastically. I remember the first time I had what was to become a common headache. My husband was going to go ride a horse, and I was home alone. All of a sudden it was like a knife sticking into my forehead. Though that headache was quite debilitating, I didn't think too much about it. However, when the headaches kept recurring, I decided I had to do something. The light hurt my eyes, and so I'd go to bed and put a pillow over my head until the headache went away. Sometimes the pain would get so intense I'd get sick. One time while driving, I suddenly needed to stick my head out of the window. (I figured it was easier to clean the outside of the truck than the inside!) I hate telling this, but that is how severe my headaches can be.

"I'm finding as I travel across the country with my evangelist husband that many, many ladies suffer with symptoms associated with something that goes wrong around the age of 40. (Sometimes I think God should have cut our age in half so instead of living until 70, we would expire at 35! Now I don't *really* think that because my husband and my kids need me, but in the midst of some of these headaches, I do wonder!) Some people say, 'Well, you know, I've just got to live with these headaches. I just go to bed for three days out of the month (or every two weeks or in whatever time cycle they recur).' But I don't believe God wants me to live with headaches, so I decided to try to find out why I was getting them and then what I could do about them. I did not want to just lay down and give in to these headaches that were robbing

> If you have melted chocolate all over your hands, you're eating it too slowly!

me of several precious days every few weeks! I want to be as effective as possible for the Lord, and I don't want to just give up days where I am totally unproductive as a wife, as a mother, and as a Christian because I failed to find solutions to my health issues. Finding help has been a long journey, but I've had a good amount of success.

"For five years I've been in the middle of this experience called menopause. For five years I've been trying to find answers. I've seen improvement, but I have not found all the answers I need. Am I angry? A little bit. Am I frustrated? A whole lot! But I'm not going to give up. What happens is that we don't keep trying to find answers, but I decided to stay on this until I find answers and get results.

"I've done a lot of research and reading on this subject. I've read at least 20 books about pre-menopause, menopause, and post-menopause (and with all I've read, I figure that including the 'pre' and the 'post' I'm going to be in this menopause thing about 35 years!)

"However, with all of my reading, I have come to believe that 'natural' is the best way for me in getting relief from the symptoms of menopause. I'm not a 'natural' person in anything—you know, I like cookies, I don't eat raw beets (I eat them pickled but not raw!), and I like junk food like pizza and Cheez-Its, but for me to feel my best, I needed to go the 'natural' route.

> Menopause: the pause that does not refresh!

"Most women are aware of the fact that the FDA is now touting great concerns about the negative side effects of the common HRT (hormone replacement therapy), which includes drugs such as Premarin. Coupled with the fact that there are many helps available which do not include dangerous side effects, I decided I wanted to avoid the negative side effects of the HRTs prescribed by most medical doctors.

"I wish I had known in my thirties about the supplements my body needed. I never took vitamins—not even a one-a-day type. I felt like I was quite healthy and just didn't feel the need to take any. However, I've come to realize that one of the causes of the extent of my problems after 40 is probably based on the fact that I didn't eat healthful foods and didn't take supplements during my twenties and thirties. Listed in Appendix C on page 151 are the supplements that I began taking that have helped me tremendously.[1]

"If you are in the midst of menopause, you know that some of the symptoms of that 'time of life' cannot only be quite frustrating, but they can also be quite debilitating. I have worked to find solutions to diminish these symptoms because my family needs me to be at my best. Therefore, I am challenging you to find good medical help.

"Because my husband is an evangelist, I meet literally hundreds of women across the country. A great percentage of the women I meet who are in their forties are struggling with this phenomenon called menopause. I wish I could say that the symptoms last a few months and go away. That is not true! The fact is, I believe that the Devil is using menopause to defeat women, wreak havoc in families, and cause women not to be effective in their service for God. Because of that, I am for doing everything possible to find solutions to the problem, one of which is finding a good physician.

"There are two avenues from which to choose when finding medical help: traditional medicine, which uses drugs to treat the symptoms, and holisitic medicine, which uses a natural approach to treating medical problems. I have found that for me (and for numbers of women I have counseled across the country) the natural route has had the most helpful solutions.

"One of the most common treatments traditional medical doctors offer is prescriptions for depression. Let me beg of you not to fall into that trap. I have talked with women who have tried these medications. The anti-depressants do not solve the problem. At best, they mask the problems, and the side effects simply complicate an already complicated situation.

"A good doctor will run tests to find your hormone levels (such as progesterone, estrogen, thyroid, and so forth). Once your hormone levels have been tested, the doctor will be able to prescribe the proper amounts of those hormones which are lacking in your body. While traditional doctors usually prescribe drugs such as Premarin, holistic physicians usually prescribe natural or bioidentical hormones such as progesterone.

"Finding a physician who can help you can be a real challenge. I have been to a number of physicians before finding a doctor who could help me. It was discouraging at times, but I needed the help, and I was determined to get it. I have been to eight different doctors. That's a lot of first-time visits!

"One doctor charged me $129 to ask me some questions and then told me, 'You're going to be okay.' She gave me no solutions! I went to another physician and said, 'I do not want to live with the symptoms of menopause.'

"His response was amazing, 'Well, the symptoms usually only last about ten years.' That's over 10 percent of my life!

"I responded, 'But I don't want to live with these symptoms for ten years. I think there must be a way I can get over them.'

"He said, 'Well, I don't know how you can get over them.' He actually told me that!

"I have spent $3,000 trying to find help. That is a lot of money. We did not have $3,000 up front, but my husband and I decided that we wanted to find solutions, and so we have made payments—sometimes $100 a month, sometimes $50, and sometimes $25— whatever we were able to pay. I'd rather make those payments on something that is helping me be a better wife and mother, than

> I gave up jogging for my health when my thighs kept rubbing together and setting my pantyhose on fire.

to save money and be sharp with my tongue and moody in my attitudes in my home. My husband and children can't take it when I'm witchy. (My family thinks a new woman moved into the house five years ago!) Sometimes I'll ask, 'Do you remember when I was nice?'

"Joe is only 11, and he'll teasingly say, 'No, Mom, I don't remember that time.' We now have fun with it. Actually, I think God has a great sense of humor since He gives menopausal women teenage girls!

"After going to seven doctors and not getting help, I found a doctor who sat down with me and asked me a lot of questions. He really listened and heard what I was saying. He ordered tests to find my hormone levels and then prescribed

bioidentical hormones for me. I am not back to my pre-menopausal self physically, but I have seen tremendous improvement in my health with the natural hormones.

"Again, let me encourage you to find a doctor who will help you with your symptoms. You're worth it; your family needs you; and God deserves to have you at your best in order to serve Him!"[2]

I agree wholeheartedly with Loretta. Do what it takes to find the help you need in order to get back on track! You are worth it, and God wants it for you!

Please note that in addition to the supplements listed in Appendix C, you will find the information to help you locate a holisitic physician on page 150 in Appendix B.

Every time I get the urge to exercise, I lie down till the feeling passes.

Opposition to Good Health

Though it is God's will for most of us to be in good health so we are able to accomplish the plans He has for our lives, we can rest assured that the Devil does not want us or any other Christian's fulfilling those plans and purposes!

When we are born, the Devil's first plan is to keep us from getting saved. When that fails and we trust Christ as our Saviour, he is forced to change his plan. His will then changes to rendering us ineffective for Christ. He wants us to do *nothing* of eternal value and immediately begins his work to defeat us. He has many methods to his madness, but one of the greatest attacks the Devil makes on Christians is on their health. He attacks our bodies. He wants us to be in poor health to lessen our effectiveness for Christ and our ability to serve Him.

Someone said to me one day, "Why do you think so many Christians are sick?" The person went on to say that it seems that a greater percentage of Christians are sick and in ill health than the unsaved. Whether that is true or not, I do not know—especially since everyone eventually dies! I have no facts on which to base that assumption. However, I do know that the Devil is very interested in thwarting our work for God. If he can get us not to take proper care of our bodies, then he is another step closer toward his goal of keeping us from being able to follow God's plan and will for our lives.

It is interesting to me that some of the most health-conscious people in our country are the "New-Age" folks. These are people whose philosophies are completely anti-God. They believe every individual is his own God (capital "G"), and they look forward to a time when a "Christ" (not Jesus Christ our Saviour) will rule the world and we will all be "one." So it is no surprise to me that many of those involved in the New-Age movement are health-conscious individuals. The Devil wants his crowd healthy, energetic, and ready to do his work. He knows his time is short and wants his forces healthy and able to do as much damage and destruction as possible.

He wants the exact opposite for Christians. He *always* wants the opposite of what God wants on every issue. The Devil is a deceiver. He wants you to believe that your physical lifestyle doesn't matter. He wants you to believe that sickness comes to everyone and that the physical maladies you begin to experience as you age (starting even as early as a person's twenties and thirties) are just part of the aging process and that there is nothing you can do about it. He wants you to believe it's all "in your genes" and that you are helpless to fight the symptoms and the poor health conditions you face.

I believe that another part of the Devil's plan involves millions of dollars' being needlessly spent each year by Christians on surgeries, medications, and doctor's appointments that could be prevented or healed by some basic lifestyle changes. It seems there is a vast amount of money that could be sent to missions and used to win souls to Christ that is being spent on surgeries, medication, and other medical needs. The Devil has blinded us and deceived us into thinking this is how it has to be.

I have nothing against the medical community. I believe most medical personnel are in their chosen career because they care about people and want to help them. *This book is not an attack on the medical community. Neither is it a declaration stating that we should never go to doctors. I am for the medical community, and I am for going to a doctor when it is necessary.*

Let me give you an example in my own life. In 2005 I fell and tore my rotator cuff in my shoulder. The pain was excruciating, and it became so bad I could not lift my arm but just a few inches. I could not raise my arm high enough to fix my hair each morning. (That's when I decided I had to do something! Anyone who's ever seen me in the morning before I curl my hair would tell you that it's scary!)

Because I knew that people often have surgery for a torn rotator cuff, my husband and I decided I should go to a major medical center for treatment. I grew up in Minnesota and am very familiar with Mayo Clinic, so I went to Rochester, Minnesota, to have my shoulder checked. I saw an orthopedic surgeon, Dr. Sperling. He did a number of rotations and movements to test my shoulder and agreed that, indeed, I did have a torn rotator cuff. I expected him to say I needed surgery; rather, he gave me a prescription for six weeks of physical therapy and told me to come back in six to eight weeks if I was not better.

I asked, "Are you going to do an MRI?" His response surprised me.

"No, I can tell by the range-of-motion tests I have done that you have a torn rotator cuff," he explained. "An MRI would be pointless at this time because it will not change the protocol for your injury. We may as well save your insurance company the expense." I was impressed! One of the aspects of Mayo Clinic we like is their conservative treatment. Surgery is a last resort rather than a first option.

> The Garlic Diet:
> You don't lose weight; you just look thinner from a distance!

34

I have a friend who is a physical therapist at St. Mary's Hospital in Rochester; she showed me the exercises I needed to do. So, rather than go to physical therapy immediately, each day I very diligently did the exercises that she had demonstrated at home. (Had that not worked, I would have gone to physical therapy as Dr. Sperling had instructed.) I also went online and learned a few additional exercises I could do. Because of this, my husband and I were able to save the cost of physical therapy. In addition to faithfully doing the prescribed exercises, I also did some research of my own and found a few additional therapies (such as a deep tissue rub) that were said to help a torn rotator cuff. In about four weeks my shoulder was completely healed, and I've had no more problem with it.

All of that to say, I am very grateful I had the medical community when I had that injury. I needed them. Had my shoulder not healed, I would probably have needed surgery because I could not function well with not being able to lift my arm more than a few inches. But I chose to seek medical help at a clinic which has a reputation for being conservative in their treatment. I also chose to find and institute some additional therapies on my own (taking responsibility for my own well being). The entire cost was about $1,020 at Mayo Clinic.

I was thrilled that God had led my husband and me in the decision-making processes and that thousands of dollars were saved (in addition to the fact that I now have full use of my shoulder which probably would not be if I'd had surgery) as a result. In the end, it saved both us and our insurance company thousands of dollars. We were able to put the money we saved toward missions and the Lord's work.

Let me say once again, I am not bashing the medical community in any way. I am simply saying that the medical community does not have the burden for my personal health and well being in the same manner that I do. So, while I consult the medical community and sometimes need their care, I cannot justify completely turning over my health and well being to them as I believe I did for a number of years. I must take personal responsibility.

First Corinthians 9:27 says, *"But I keep under my body, and bring it into subjection: lest that by any means, when I have preached to others, I myself should be a castaway."* It is interesting that the word *body* appears 44 times in the book of I Corinthians. Though every use of the word does not apply to our physical body, many do. This is a book that was written to the Corinthian people—a very undisciplined group of Christians who lived much of their lives by the lust of the flesh. God expects us to be disciplined with our bodies, and He expects us to take care of our bodies. The care and

> "I told my doctor I get very tired when I go on a diet, so he gave me pep pills. Know what happened? I ate faster."
> – Joe E. Lewis

welfare of my body is my responsibility.

Second Corinthians 5:10 says, *"For we must all appear before the judgment seat of Christ; that every one may receive the things done in his body, according to that he hath done, whether it be good or bad."* God expects us to be good stewards of the body He has given us. The care of my body is my responsibility.

Acts 10:38 says, *"How God anointed Jesus of Nazareth with the Holy Ghost and with power: who went about doing good, and healing all that were oppressed of the devil; for God was with him."* Now, I am not a "spooky" Christian, nor do I think Christianity is "spooky." I am not one of those people who is into big discussions about people's being demon possessed, oppressed, etc. I believe

Say Something Positive

A husband and wife were getting ready for bed. The wife stood in front of a full-length mirror taking a hard look at herself. "You know, Dear," she said, "I look in the mirror, and I see an old woman. My face is all wrinkled, my hair is grey, my shoulders are hunched over, I've got fat legs, and my arms are all flabby." She turned to her husband and said, "Tell me something positive to make me feel better about myself."

He studied hard for a moment thinking about it and then said in a soft, thoughtful voice, "Well, there's nothing wrong with your eyesight."

that the Word of God is very practical for our everyday lives. This verse says that Jesus *healed* those who were *oppressed* of the Devil. The word *healed* means, "to cure, make well." *Oppressed* means, "to use one's power against one." I believe that this verse demonstrates clearly that the Devil wants to defeat us in the area of our health.

I don't believe we need to spend hours thinking on the fact that the Devil is trying to fight our good health. Nor do I think we need to constantly be giving him credit for our poor health. I don't like giving him attention any more than I like giving a naughty child attention for things he does to get his way. However, I do think it is important to realize that the fight for our health is more than just a physical battle. We are in a spiritual warfare, and to understand that helps us understand more fully that we cannot fight this battle alone!

Ephesians 6:11–13 says, *"Put on the whole armour of God, that ye may be able to stand against the wiles* [craftily framed devices, to deceive] *of the devil. For we wrestle not against flesh and blood, but against principalities, against powers, against the rulers of the darkness of this world, against spiritual wickedness in high places. Wherefore take unto you the whole armour of God, that ye may be able to withstand in the evil day, and having done all, to stand."* As you face your struggle with poor health and try to implement changes, please keep in mind that you must take the *"whole armour of God"* with you and use it in order to see real, lasting victory and healing.

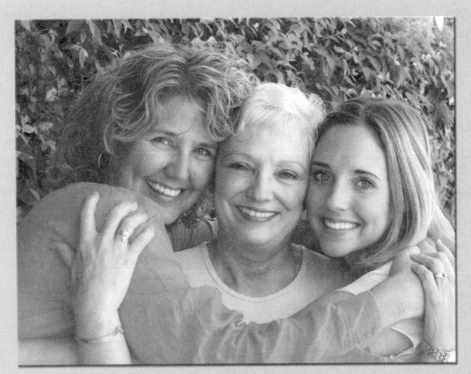

PART THREE

The Body
and How It Works

The Goal: A Healthy Metabolism

Because I want to help you better understand the wonderful body God created and have a foundational knowledge of how it works, this unit is more factual than practical. I've tried to simplify the facts, but if you don't comprehend it on your first reading, I would encourage you to read it several times so you get a better understanding of your metabolism. (It took many "reads" and much study for me to finally get this, so if you get it the first time, you can mark your intellect at the genius level!)

God designed a phenomenal "machine" when He created the human body. It is a very complex creation with remarkable systems—a "well-oiled machine" if you will. We truly are fearfully and wonderfully made! *"I will praise thee; for I am fearfully and wonderfully made: marvellous are thy works; and that my soul knoweth right well."* (Psalm 139:14)

A healthy body requires a healthy metabolism. The word *metabolism* conjures up different meanings for different people, but for most of us, it simply indicates the rate at which we burn calories. (And for most of us, that's not fast enough!) Because that mind set leads to wrong thinking on weight control, let me explain the metabolism.

God designed our bodies to stay alive and to function with biochemicals. These biochemicals are used for *structure, function,* and *energy*. Listed in the box below are some examples of each.

Structural Biochemicals: organs, glands, cells, teeth, hair, skin, nails, muscles, bones, connective tissues (the physical makeup of our bodies)
Functional Biochemicals: neuro-transmitters, enzymes, hormones, antibodies (those things which send messages and cause our bodies to function)
Energy Biochemicals: sugar, ketones, triglycerides, glycogen (those things which give our bodies the energy to function)

These biochemicals undergo continuous chemical reactions in order to carry out all of the body's functions. For example, for your heart to beat, you must have a heart (structural biochemical), signals to your heart to beat (functional biochemical), and energy to contract the muscles of the heart to cause the heartbeat (energy biochemical).

This type of reaction occurs thousands of times every day throughout your body, whether it is voluntary (you choose to do it—such as talk, eat, walk, etc.) or involuntary (those actions that happen without conscious involvement—heartbeat, breathing, digestive processes, and so forth). Every time we breathe, think, ride a bike, read a book, eat a meal, or perform *any* other activity throughout the day, we use up some of each of the three types of biochemicals.

As they are used, all of these cells must be replaced. We must rebuild the same biochemicals we have used so we can perform these same activities again. The using up followed by the rebuilding of biochemicals is called **regeneration.**

The sum total of all of these regenerations—the using-up followed by the building-up reactions—is known as your **metabolism**. An efficient or healthy metabolism causes all of these chemical reactions to occur on a continuous basis where our bodies rebuild as many biochemicals as we use. Quite simply put, we are constantly using up cells which must be replaced. *The process of using up and replacing those cells is called our metabolism.* Metabolism is the continuous chemical and physical process in living cells including the changing of food into living tissue and the changing of living tissue into waste products and energy.

> The older you get, the tougher it is to lose weight because by then, your body and your fat are really good friends.

There are two parts to the metabolism cycle: the using-up side and the building-up side. For optimum health, these two parts must be kept in balance. When you provide the nutrition, the rest, and the healthful lifestyle your metabolism needs, your body turns into an efficiently running machine. Allow me to compare the metabolism to a steam engine.

My dad was a farmer who worked hard and had little time for play. He did, however, have one hobby. When I was in third grade, he purchased a four-passenger Cessna airplane. Initially he used it to travel from Illinois where we lived to Minnesota where he was looking to buy a farm. He did buy a farm in Minnesota, and we moved there on Ground Hogs Day in 1962 when I was 11 years old. After the move he kept his plane, and occasionally, at the end of a hard day's work, he would clean up and take some of us up for a ride.

When Dad was about 65, he was diagnosed with a heart condition that prevented him from being able to renew his pilot's license. He took one last flight in that airplane and then sold it. With the money from the plane, he purchased a 1901 Minneapolis steam engine that had originally been used to thrash grain early in the twentieth century. When my siblings or I would come for a visit, one of his requests was often, "Would you 'fire up' the steam engine?"

We, of course, were happy to oblige and would fill the firebox with wood and the boiler with water. We'd start a fire in the wood box and wait for the water to boil. When the water began to boil, the steam engine would begin to run. It was a smooth, almost melodic sound. The rhythmic "tcha, tcha, tcha" of the engine always brought a smile to Dad's face. He liked to just sit and listen to that sound (and, of course, several of us, like my sister Joan and I, especially enjoyed blowing the whistle!) Dad could sit and enjoy the workings and sound of the steam engine for several hours at a time. It was well maintained and really was a well-oiled machine. When we placed the proper elements into the steam engine which it needed to make it run, it ran very smoothly. Though my dad used it simply for enjoyment, it was originally designed and built to perform a heavy work load for farmers.

Our bodies are also built to work. As long as we keep them maintained and put the proper ingredients into our bodies, they will work like the "well-oiled machine" they were made to be. What would have happened if we had put wood in the wood box of the steam engine and lit it, but we failed to put any water in the boiler? We would have caused some major damage to the boiler and to the steam engine. Wouldn't it have been ridiculous to get frustrated at the steam engine if we put water in the boiler but no wood in the firebox? Yet, we mistreat our bodies and then wonder why we have gained weight, why we are so tired all the time, or why we have diseases such as cancer or diabetes.

Patients are often told regarding diseases from which they are suffering, "It's genetic." Though there is a definite connection with our genes and which *type* of diseases we eventually face, it is the damage we do at the cellular level to our metabolism that actually causes the diseases. Yes, unless we make some wise choices and make the necessary lifestyle changes that will heal our metabolism or keep it healthy in the first place, we are destined to repeat the same health issues our parents and our grandparents faced—and often at a much younger age; however, the diseases come because we fail to take care of the "machine," not because Grandma and Grandpa had coronary heart disease or some other chronic health issue!

While the body is continually involved in the using up of cells, a serious imbalance is caused when we fail to provide the necessary tools the body must have to efficiently rebuild the cells it has used. Since every system and function of the body is connected, your metabolism is only as efficient as your chemical reactions (regeneration). Inefficient regeneration— hence an *unhealthy metabolism*—causes your body to get out of balance. The result over time is disease, obesity, and a myriad of health problems. The longer the body's regener-

> Skinny people make me mad, especially when they say things like, "You know, sometimes I forget to eat." Now, I've forgotten my address, my mother's maiden name, and my keys. But I've *never* forgotten to eat.

ation is inefficient, the more unhealthy a person's metabolism becomes, and the longer it takes to regain a healthy metabolism. Failing to properly rebuild the cells that are used up leads to disease, obesity, and fatigue. Not only does it lead to obesity, it leads to a *disproportionate weight gain* in specific areas of the body, especially the mid-section.

Take the quiz below to learn the state of your metabolism. Place an "x" in each box beside the symptoms that apply to you.

Metabolism Evaluation Quiz

☐ Lack of energy
☐ Poor memory and difficulty concentrating
☐ Mood swings
☐ Poor sleep habits
☐ Poor digestion and elimination
☐ Lack of strength
☐ Weak bones, teeth, hair, and nails
☐ Addictions (including refined sugars, artificial sweeteners, caffeine, nicotine, alcohol, or drugs)
☐ Chronic unexplained pain, allergies, asthma, frequent severe headaches, frequent heartburn, frequent infections
☐ Degenerative diseases of aging such as cancer, heart disease, high blood pressure, obesity, osteoarthritis, osteoporosis, stroke, type II diabetes, abnormal cholesterol levels, early menopause

_____ **Total number of boxes checked**

Interpreting your Results:

- 0 — Very Healthy Metabolism
- 1–2 — Fairly Healthy Metabolism
- 3 or more of the first 7 **or** if you checked number 8 or 9 — Damaged Metabolism
- If you checked number 10 — Badly Damaged Metabolism[1]

If this quiz was "bad news" for you, let me give you some good news. You can help your metabolism to heal! Remember, your metabolism is not just the rate at which you burn calories; rather, your metabolism is how efficiently and how effectively you build up and replace the cells you have used. That is why attaining and maintaining proper weight control is not as simple as just cutting calories. The common mind set today is that one should lose weight to become healthy. Quite the opposite is true. ***We must become healthy (heal our metabolism) to achieve proper weight control and optimum health.***

Our goal should not be to lose weight, but to heal our metabolism. A healthy metabolism will take care of the weight problem and other health issues you are experiencing The metabolism is a very complex series of the chemical reactions which are affected by a person's lifestyle. Medical research has shown that regaining a

> Chocolate-covered raisins, cherries, orange slices, and strawberries all count as fruit, so eat as many as you want.

healthy metabolism involves five major issues
which will each be discussed at length in Part IV:

- Proper intake and output (eating, drinking, and elimination)
- Proper emotional and physical stress management
- Proper exercise, sunlight, and oxygen
- Proper elimination of toxic chemicals
- Proper bioidentical hormone replacement

The Problem:
How to get two
pounds of
chocolate home
from the store
in a hot car.

The Solution:
Eat it in the
parking lot.

What Causes a Damaged Metabolism?

A damaged metabolism occurs when your lifestyle choices tell the body to "use up" without also providing the means for it to regenerate. Your body cannot continue to use up and use up without regenerating and remain healthy! A damaged metabolism is brought on by mistakes we make in lifestyle choices. Fad diets rank up at the top! This would include low-calorie diets, low-fat diets, high protein diets, low-carb diets, etc. The problem with these fad diets is that they deprive your body of nutrition it desperately needs.

Another cause of a damaged metabolism is skipping meals (usually breakfast and/or lunch) or fasting to try to lose weight. Skipping meals and not eating wreaks havoc with your metabolism because, once again, it deprives your body of the nutrients it needs.

Other causes of a damaged metabolism include excessive exercise, lack of sleep, poor nutritional choices, stress, ingesting toxic chemicals, and failing to properly address hormone deficiencies.

To help you understand how you most likely damaged your metabolism (and therefore have experienced weight gain, illness, or fatigue...or all three!), check the following habits that have been a part of your life:

- ☐ Skipping meals
- ☐ Not eating enough carbohydrates, enough proteins, and/or enough fat
- ☐ Eating too many carbohydrates, too much protein, and/or too much fat
- ☐ Emotional stress
- ☐ Chronic pain
- ☐ Not sleeping enough (7 to 8 hours of uninterrupted sleep a night)
- ☐ Ingesting or using toxic chemicals such as street drugs, tobacco, alcohol, soda, diet soda, refined sugar, caffeine, and most medications
- ☐ Excessive cardiovascular exercise...or not exercising at all
- ☐ Not taking bioidentical hormone replacement therapy if needed, or taking it incorrectly[1]

We live in a weight-conscious, crazed society that is obsessed with being thin. That obsession causes people by the thousands to spend money on weight-loss books, diets, supplements, exercise equipment, and so forth. It seems that for most people, it does not matter how the goal is accomplished; the important thing is to arrive at the goal. That goal is weight loss at any cost in order to be thin.

All of this obsession with weight loss and being thin (a very lucrative business, by the way, for those who are "selling") has caused us to become a very overweight, fatigued society. It is interesting that the more we "diet" the heavier the general population becomes. The more we deprive ourselves and the harder we work to lose weight the sicker our society becomes.

How frustrating for people who once had a well-proportioned body shape to now have fat deposits which have settled around their mid-section. I met a lady who was trying on clothes in the dressing room next to mine. She walked out, looked at me (I was standing in front of the mirror) and said, "That skirt looks nice on you. My body is so out of proportion I can't even get skirts to look decent on me any more. They hang funny." She went on to say, "I weighed 102 and was a size 4 until I hit 40. Now look at me. It's all around here," as she pointed to her mid-section and hip area.

She is a beautiful woman who is experiencing what

> **Diet Tip**
> Eat a chocolate bar before each meal. It will take the edge off your appetite, and you'll eat less!

numbers of other women all across America are experiencing. She has gone from a size 4 to probably about a size 20 or 22 and can't seem to find answers. I did not get into a "women's health" discussion with her and ask all about her history, but one thing is for sure, I did perceive that the lady has a damaged metabolism. However, she is not helpless and hopeless. There are answers for her and for other ladies with the same symptoms.

The problem is that most people are looking for a "quick fix." I have women tell me on a regular basis, "I know this diet probably isn't the best for me, but I just want to get the weight off. Then I'll worry about my eating habits." What they don't realize is that to go on another fad diet is to take another step toward further damaging their metabolism. At some point our bodies rebel and say, "No more!" It is then that we can't seem to lose weight even on the fad diets! Fad diets are a short-term fix that signal "use up" to the body disproportionately to signaling "rebuild." Using up and using up and using up without rebuilding at the same rate is going to damage your metabolism. The more this happens, the more damaged one's metabolism becomes. There is no arguing with the fact that fad diets do usually get the weight off for a while. The problem is that they cause such terrible damage to the metabolism in the process.

While the common philosophy is, "I'm going to lose weight so I can become healthy," the exact opposite is true. Dr. Diana Schwarzbein, author of the book, *The Schwarzbein Principle—The Program*, a book on losing weight the healthy way, states repeatedly, "You need to be healthy to lose weight, not lose weight to be healthy."[2] Let me explain:

1. An overweight person has ill health *because* of a damaged metabolism. A person cannot properly lose weight or regain broken health without first healing the metabolism.

2. The metabolism will never be healed by continuing the habits that damaged it in the first place. (i.e. poor nutrition, lack of sleep, etc.)

3. The root problems must be addressed to heal the metabolism.

4. Once the metabolism is healed, the body will be able to lose the excess and unwanted weight. A healthy metabolism will also help your body structure to return to its proper proportion giving you a more balanced body shape.

5. Just as it has taken years to wear down your body and damage your metabolism, it takes time to rebuild your body and to heal your metabolism.

It is important to understand that your health—a healthy metabolism—is the important issue, not how much you weigh! Once your metabolism is healthy, your body is then able to shed those excess pounds! Rather than concentrating on losing weight, concentrate on breaking the bad habits that caused the excess weight—a damaged metabolism! Remember, you do not have a "fast" or a "slow" metabolism. You either have a "healthy" or "damaged" metabolism.

Thin Does Not Equal Healthy!

Just because a person is thin does not mean she has a healthy metabolism. She may be thin but have a myriad of other problems such as fatigue, cancer, arthritis, diabetes, Alzheimer's, etc. Whether it is obesity, degenerative diseases, or fatigue, the problem is a damaged metabolism.

It is also important to realize that a person does not damage her metabolism overnight. It was a process that happened over a number of years. Therefore, the repair does not happen overnight. This is a process that takes time. It has taken a lot longer than I have wanted to see the healing I have experienced, but the better I feel and the more understanding I have gained, the less I am tempted to quit and go back to my old habits.

The road to good health is a journey. Realize it will take time—which is really the best way to change anything in your life. Deuteronomy 7:22 says, *"And the LORD thy God will put out those nations before thee by little and little: thou mayest not consume them at once, lest*

> **Queen Size**
> A little boy went to the store with his grandmother, and on the way home, he looked at the things she had purchased. He found a package of panty hose and began to sound out the words "QUEEN SIZE." He then turned to his grandmother and exclaimed, "Look, Granny, you wear the same size as our bed!"

the beasts of the field increase upon thee." God knew it would be much better for the Israelites to win the battles one step at a time than to have "instant victory."

Growth in the Christian life is not instant. People who grow too rapidly are not able to maintain the changes they make. It is much better to make one change and get that "under your belt" so to speak than to make a number of changes too quickly that you do not have the character to maintain. You want the changes to become a way of life (a habit). Habits take time to form. *Take the time it takes to make one change at a time to make it a permanent change—a habit—in your life.*

In other words, heal your metabolism one change at a time!

Question:
Why is there no such organization as "Chocoholics Anonymous"?

Answer:
Because no one wants to quit!

Hello! Can You Hear Me Now?

A particular cell phone company at one time had an advertisement where an employee calls the home office from all different out-of-the-way places to make sure the relay towers are giving strong, clear signals and that the messages are getting through. The employee constantly asks the question, "Can you hear me now?"

Just as cell phones must have a clear signal so their operators can hear each other, our bodies have must have strong, clear signals also to be sure the proper messages are relayed from the cells to the different body systems. The "messengers" in our bodies are hormones. The metabolic system (your "metabolism") is completely dependent upon the correct messages' getting through to each of the body systems. It seems that many of us have hormones saying to our body systems, "Can you hear me now?" The answer is "No!" because our hormones are out of balance and the proper messages are not getting through.

I believe hormones are another one of those misunderstood parts of the metabolic process. Just as I always thought that the metabolism was simply how fast my body burned the calories I took

in, I have always thought of hormones simply as some part of the reproductive process. I never realized that *every* body system operates by hormones.

So, what exactly are hormones? **Hormones are chemical messengers secreted into blood or extracellular fluid by one cell that affect the functioning of other cells.**

Most hormones circulate in blood, coming into contact with essentially all cells. However, a given hormone usually affects only a limited number of cells, which are called **target cells**.

Hormone receptors are found either exposed on the surface of the cell or within the cell, depending on the type of hormone. In very basic terms, when a particular hormone binds to a receptor, it triggers a cascade of reactions within the cell that affects function.

Our bodies have a system of glands called the endocrine system which produce substances called hormones. These "chemical messengers" are released into the bloodstream, go to their target cells, and influence them to act in a specific way or carry out a specific function.

Every cell has a receptor enabling it to be influenced by a specific hormone. As stated previously, hormones are the "messenger boys" that give instructions to the cells. So as the hormones traffic throughout the body they come into contact with many different cells. However, only the cells that have the specific receptor for a particular hormone is targeted by and responds to that hormone. The specific cells for each hormone are called target cells— cells which have the receptor for that particular hormone. Cells which do not contain a receptor for a particular hormone cannot be influenced directly by that hormone.

Reception of a radio broadcast provides a good analogy. Everyone within range of a transmitter for National Public Radio is exposed to that signal (even if they don't contribute!). However, in order to be a National Public Radio target and thus influenced directly by their broadcasts, you must have a receiver tuned to that frequency.

Hormone receptors are found either exposed on the surface of the cell or within the cell, depending on the type of hormone. In very basic terms, when a particular hormone binds to a receptor, it triggers a cascade of reactions within the cell that affects function.[1]

Example: insulin is a hormone secreted by the pancreas. When carbohydrates are consumed, the pancreas is notified that sugar is hitting the blood stream. Insulin is then released into the bloodstream to control blood-sugar levels. (Without insulin our blood-sugar levels would get so high we would die.)

Hormones are responsible for breaking down old cells and rebuilding new ones. Those healthy new cells are important for hormone production. In turn, those hormones are responsible for breaking down old cells and rebuilding new ones, which in turn produce more hormones. On and on the cycle goes.

When any one hormonal system breaks down, it affects all the other processes in the entire physiological system because every system in the body is interconnected. For the body to function properly and at optimum, all hormones must be kept at normal levels. That is when we experience the best health and the most energy.

When hormones are not at normal levels, we experience fatigue, disease, etc. For example, a high carbohydrate diet causes prolonged high insulin levels (imbalance). High insulin levels in turn disrupt other hormone levels and cause, among other things, an imbalance in cholesterol

> Put "eat chocolate" at the top of your list of things to do today. That way, at least you'll get one thing done.

levels which can lead to heart problems, strokes, etc.

Now, what is a key to balanced hormonal levels? On what are hormones dependent for normal production and function? Fats and proteins! Hormones are made from and regulated by the protein and fat that we eat.

For a number of years there has been a media barrage of "low-fat" hype. However, fat is not our enemy! Fat is our friend and is necessary for healthy cell membranes. It also plays a vital role in the production of hormones.

Eating fat does not make us fat. Rather, eating healthful fats actually enables us to heal our metabolism which helps us to lose weight more effectively as well as rid our bodies of diseases caused by a damaged metabolism. (Please don't put this book down to run out and order a quarter-pounder with cheese and large fries! The *types* of fat you eat are as important as the eating of fat!)

In order to have a balanced system, we must replenish the resources and energy stores for all the cellular processes in the body. When we fail to do so, we signal our body that we are starving (In actuality, our cells are starving for the nutrients they need to tear down and rebuild.) Our metabolism becomes less efficient, and we gain weight. A person who is overweight is a person whose hormones are out of balance.

When we do not eat the necessary proteins and fats for cellular maintenance, our bodies adapt. For example, protein, fat, and normal hormone levels are needed to make hair. When you do not eat the required nutrients and do not have normal hormone levels, the body will use its own protein such as bones or hair. That is why a person with a thyroid imbalance or other hormonal imbalances such as a lack of progesterone often has thinning hair. (I am not referring to baldness which is generally a genetic condition.)

While hormones are the key to a healthy metabolism, eating a balanced diet will help keep your hormones in balance. Eating the proper foods will keep the signals moving efficiently and clearly through the body. When your hormones say, "Can you hear me now?" the body systems should be able to answer quickly and clearly, "Yes, we can!"

Prayers Before Eating

The Sunday school teacher asked, "Now, Johnny, tell me, do you say prayers before eating?"

"No, Sir," little Johnny replied, "I don't have to. My mom is a good cook."

Keeping Your Age and the Aging Process in Balance

Aging is a result of a "breakdown of the building side of your metabolic system—the inability of your body to regenerate itself fast enough to recover from the wear and tear of everyday life."[1]

Psalm 90:10 says, *"The days of our years are threescore years and ten; and if by reason of strength they be fourscore years, yet is their strength labour and sorrow; for it is soon cut off, and we fly away."* This verse teaches that basically God gives each of us threescore and ten (70) years to live. Our body's rebuilding ability decreases as we age. That process is called "metabolic aging."

Each of us has a good amount of control over the rate of our metabolic aging. Statistics say that 35 percent is genetic. In other words, we have control of 65 percent of the condition of our health. The more abuses our bodies experience—those habits which damage our metabolism—the faster we age and the sooner we begin to experience degenerative diseases (and the sooner we die). Our lifestyle choices can either increase or decrease the aging process in our bodies, which thereby determines how long we live along with our quality of life while we are alive.

I was delivering a birthday gift to a lady for someone, and I said cheerfully, "So, how old are you today?"

She said, "Old enough" letting me know she does not tell her age.

Her sister-in-law was with her and said, "I don't hide my age. I'm 64." I could not believe she was 64. I actually thought she was younger than I am. I had never met these ladies before, but my guess is that the 64-year-old lady has lived a basically moderate lifestyle. From all appearances, she seems to be healthy. She appears to have been good to her body.

While women are sometimes known for being concerned about their physical age and for not wanting to tell how old they are, their real concern should be their metabolic age. Are we making lifestyle choices to slow down the aging process (and all of the diseases and frustrations that go with it)? The healthier our metabolism, the younger—the more "in balance"—our bodies are.

The best 10 years of a woman's life are between 39 and 40.

Because we live in a society obsessed with "thin," it is very difficult to get beyond the weight-loss issues we face. It's as if losing the weight will take care of all the other problems. I want to re-emphasize that our main goal should not be weight loss. Our main goal should be a healthy metabolism. Why? A healthy metabolism will not only enable us to take off the weight we need to lose, it will also care for the other problems we face such as fatigue, chronic diseases, pain, and so forth. You cannot properly lose weight and keep it off if you have an unhealthy metabolism. If you use "quick-fix" type measures (such as fad diets) to get your weight off, you will simply do more damage to your metabolism and face more health issues, obesity, and fatigue down the road.

The less damaged your metabolism is when you start making important lifestyle changes, the faster you will recover your energy, your health, and the faster you will reach your ideal weight and body shape. Conversely, the more damaged your metabolism and the worse condition your body is in, the longer it will take to heal. You cannot change what you've done in the past. Nor can you magically change the state of your metabolism today. To whatever degree your metabolism is damaged, it is done, but the choices you make from this point on help deter-

> How old would you be if you didn't know how old you are? "Old is an attitude!"

mine the future health of your metabolism.

Let me plead with you to put aside all the "quick fixes" and the fad diets which are so tempting to someone who is overweight. Decide today that you are going to make the *lifestyle changes* you need to make to recover your health.

Also decide that no matter how difficult or long the struggle, you are going to stick with the principles that will add years and effectiveness to your life.

Please take note that when a person's metabolism is very damaged, it is not uncommon for that person to gain weight while the metabolism is healing before losing weight once the metabolism is well on its way to being repaired. Decide up front that no matter what the struggles, you are going to stick with the principles to heal your metabolism! It will be well worth the effort and the struggle!

I want you to also keep in mind that I am praying for you. I believe this is a serious matter because this struggle is a spiritual warfare. The Devil wants your health. He wants to deprive you of good years serving God.

Why don't you put this book aside for a few minutes, get down on your knees, and ask God to help you in this struggle. You can pray your own prayer, or you may use the example at the end of this chapter. You may want to write this prayer (or one similar to it) in your prayer journal or on a 3x5 card and place it in your Bible with your Bible reading schedule so you see it every day. I think it would be wise for you to pray this prayer every day. Include God in every part of your struggle! He's where the victory is.

I also suggest you find a Bible verse to claim as God's promise to bring healing to your metabolism as you institute His principles. Memorize the Bible verse you choose and quote it often.

Dear Lord,

I realize that my struggle with poor health and weight control is both a physical battle and a spiritual battle and that the state of my health can help or hinder me in my work for eternity. I need Your help to regain my health:

- Please give me the wisdom to know lifestyle and habit changes I need to make.
- Please give me the character to make one change at a time to improve my health.
- Please give me the character I need to stick with those changes.
- Please give me the character I need to continue on with the changes no matter what obstacles or struggles come.

I love You, Jesus, and I need You. I am asking for Your help so I can serve You more, praise You more, honor You more, and be all You want me to be. Thank You for hearing me. Amen.

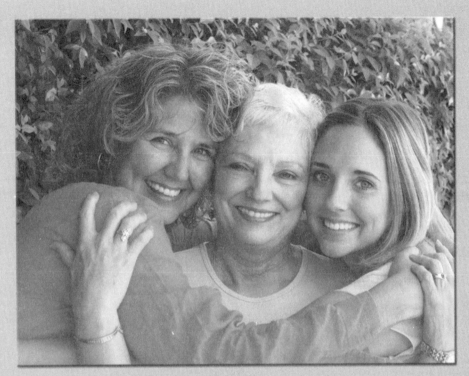

PART FOUR

Five Steps
to Good Health

The Five Steps

This unit explains five practical steps a person should institute to regain a healthy metabolism. Those steps include:

- Proper nutrition and elimination)
- Proper sleep and stress management
- Proper exercise, sunlight, and oxygen
- Proper elimination of toxic chemicals
- Proper bioidentical hormone replacement when needed

Because the single most important change you can make to restore your health is to begin eating a balanced diet, I will be addressing that issue first. Decide it is a priority to make the dietary changes you need to make as your first step toward healing your metabolism.

Make the changes as quickly as you are able to do so, but be patient with yourself. Do not let the following pages overwhelm you. Make the changes one step at a time, and when you feel you have fallen short, just get up and try again. Decide you will work at this for the long haul, not just two or three months or until you tire of the struggle.

If the results of the metabolism quiz you took earlier showed that you have a badly damaged metabolism, it is vital that you understand it is going to take some time to heal your body! Also, realize that every time you get discouraged and quit that you are simply prolonging the healing process.

Proverbs 24:16 says, *"For a just man falleth seven times, and riseth up again: but the wicked shall fall into mischief."* There is no doubt that you will fail sometimes in your struggle to regain your health. When you fail, simply claim Proverbs 24:16. The word *falleth* in reference to a just man is the idea of stumbling and getting back up. The word *fall* in reference to the wicked is "to fall and never get back up." Romans 8:37 is another wonderful promise, *"Nay, in all these things we are more than conquerors through him that loved us."* It is God's will that you conquer the things that are defeating you.

I am passionate about wanting see you restored to health, but God wants His will for you even more than I do. He is for you, and He wants to help you institute the principles that will help restore your health, your vitality, and ultimately, your service for Him.

As your health improves, I am begging that you show God your gratitude by using that renewed strength to make your life count for eternity. No doubt there will be some "catching up" to do if you have been in extremely poor health for a lengthy period of time. Just be sure God is very much a part of your life and the focus of your energies.

My purpose for writing this book is not for you to be able to get restored health and a beautiful body to make that the focus of your life. There is a particular store where I shop for clothes. The manager in the store was a pretty lady and always so helpful and friendly. She was also quite obese. Over the course of a year, I was in the store three or four times, and each time she had lost a marked amount of weight. The last time I saw her she had pictures to show me the progression of her weight loss. The pictures from each "era" got

sexier and sexier with more revealing clothes. One day she was not in, and I asked about her. I was told, "Oh, she doesn't work here anymore. She left her husband and her family and is living a pretty fast lifestyle." How sad!

What happened to this lady is not at all what I have in mind for your life, nor is it God's will. I will have failed you if I only help you regain your health, lose weight, and get a beautiful body. The whole purpose of my writing this book is to enable you to do more for eternity. Keep your focus on things eternal—whether you are tempted to quit that which will bring good health or whether you are tempted to go toward the world, wrong dress, and wrong actions because of success. This book is all about serving God and making a difference for eternity!

And now, let's get on with the program that will help you regain your health, your energy, and your life!

Nutrition

According to a recent article on nutrition, eating right doesn't have to be at all complicated. Nutritionists say there is a simple way to tell if you're eating right—colors. Fill your plates with bright colors of greens, reds, and yellows.

In fact, I did that this morning. I had an entire bowl of M&M's. It was delicious. I never knew eating right could be so easy!

Proper Nutrition and Elimination

The first important step toward healing your metabolism includes three parts:

- Eating a balanced diet
- Drinking plenty of pure water
- Proper elimination

A Balanced Diet

When I use the term "balanced diet," I am not speaking of "going on a diet." The term *diet* gives the idea of a short-term fix for being overweight. What happens with most people when they go on a "diet" is that they change their eating choices for a while to get weight off. When they reach their target weight, they go back to their former habits…unless they get discouraged first and stop the plan before reaching their goal.

What is needed is not a "diet" but a "lifestyle" of healthful habits. The most important step you can take to regain your health and to heal your metabolism is to eat *real foods* to give your body the nourishment it needs to rebuild the cells it uses up each day. *Real* foods as opposed to processed and man-made foods are those foods God made for us to eat such as fruits, vegetables, grain, fish, and meat.

I have talked with ladies who have consistently stayed at their desired weight for most or all of their adult life. These are also ladies who have few health issues. For years I told myself that most ladies who maintain their desired weight do so because they have a "fast" metabolism. I also told myself, "Those ladies don't have a clue about weight control; they just haven't struggled as I have."

How WRONG I was!! As I have talked with these ladies, I have found that my assumptions were very mistaken. I have yet to hear one of them say, "I pretty much eat what I want. I have a terrible time gaining weight." Quite the opposite is true. Every lady with whom I have talked has told me she has had to discipline her food choices throughout her adult life and that her struggle increased when she hit her forties. These ladies have paid a price to have good health and maintain proper weight control.

I chose to talk with ladies known as balanced, victorious Christians who live their lives by Biblical principles. It is interesting that a key element in their lifestyle choices is balance. Luke 2:52 says, *"And Jesus increased in wisdom and stature, and in favour with God and man."* In other words, Jesus was a very balanced Person.

While one of the common denominators in ladies who maintain proper weight control and good health is that of eating a balanced, nutritional diet, I am finding a common denominator in women who are overweight or in poor health—a lack of knowledge as to what it means to eat a balanced diet.

Nearly every magazine on the newsstands advertises articles on dieting. These diets run the gamut from low-fat, high-carb diets to high-protein, low-carb diets, and everything in between. All of this propaganda regarding food choices has led to great confusion.

Lorraine Day, a health oriented physician who made drastic dietary changes and who has recovered from breast cancer says, "Every disease is caused by malnutrition." In other words, diseases come because we are not providing the nutrients our cells need to rebuild each day. So, what is a balanced diet?

A balanced diet consists of:

- Three meals of *real* food a day along with one or two smaller meals (snacks) a day, each of which include real foods from the four basic food groups.
- The four food groups include: protein, fats, non-starchy vegetables, and real or complex carbohydrates.

Because each of these food groups has a specific job in rebuilding and maintaining our bodies, we need to eat foods from all of these groups at each meal every day. Real foods are foods God provides through nature—from the plant and animal kingdoms. Man-made foods are processed foods that are damaged and filled with toxic chemicals.

Eating a balanced diet from the four food groups does not mean that you will eat the same amount of food from each group. I will give you guidelines as I explain each food group to help you know portion sizes for each meal. (Note: In Appendix A on page 145 you will find charts that list foods from each of the four food groups along with guidelines to help you in making wise nutritional choices for each of your meals.)

"I've been on a constant diet for the last two decades. I've lost a total of 789 pounds. By all accounts, I should be hanging from a charm bracelet."
– Erma Bombeck

Proteins

Proteins (along with fats) are not only responsible for making bones, hair, and nails, they are also necessary for the formation of all biochemicals needed such as hormones, enzymes, and neurotransmitters. Protein steadies blood sugar and triggers the release of anti-hunger hormones. Researchers have found that protein suppresses appetite-stimulating hormones more than any other food.

Proteins include meat, poultry, fish, nuts, cheese, and vegetable proteins such as tofu. White cheeses such as mozzarella, Muenster, and goat cheese are healthier than yellow cheeses. Also, remember that nuts, cheese, and vegetable proteins also contain some carbohydrates, so you will want to limit these.

Nuts are healthiest when eaten raw as opposed to roasted. Roasted nuts usually have added salt and fat, and the roasting process reduces the nutritional value of the nuts and can damage the fat in the nuts.

Recommended Daily Protein Intake:

Advertising is a most powerful medium in our country. Of course, the whole purpose for advertising is to make money. It would be ideal if all advertising was done honestly with the complete good of the viewers in mind. Not so! The beef, pork, and chicken industries want to sell their product and want the customer to believe the body needs large servings of protein at each meal. One of the problems with serving sizes in our nation is what my friend Carol Tudor calls "portion distortion." Most of us are way out of perspective in what we think a "normal" serving size should equal.

People think nothing of consuming a 6- to 8-ounce piece of meat (or larger) at a meal. Because of improper advertising and much misinformation either directly stated or implied, people think that is what their body needs. You may be quite surprised to find that your body does not need near the amount of protein that most people consume each day.

Most adults need only about 6 *to 10 ounces of protein a day.* The average adult consumes 17 to 20 ounces of protein daily. A few years ago at Mayo Clinic, I talked with a dietician. I was shocked when she showed me the maximum amount of protein I should eat at a meal. She told me I should eat about two ounces of protein at a meal and said, "That is about one-half the size of the palm of your hand and the thickness of a deck of cards."

People who go on "high-protein" diets talk of the great amount of energy they have. No doubt that is true, but what they don't realize is that all of that protein is stimulating their adrenal glands and eventually will cause adrenal burnout which results in a damaged metabolism. Eating too much protein also causes problems such as arthritis, kidney stones, and gout—all very painful diseases. Your body does need protein—in *moderation.*

Fats

Healthy fat is needed for energy and also to rebuild your functional and structural biochemicals. Consuming healthy fats is essential to having a

> A Balanced Diet
> If I eat equal amounts of dark and white chocolate, is that a balanced diet?

healthy metabolism and a healthy body. Consuming the proper types of fat helps you feel satisfied after you have eaten (which helps to curb cravings and overeating) and also helps to build a healthy immune system.

> Vegetarian:
> Old Indian word for "Bad Hunter"

Many people believe a low-fat diet is healthy and will help them lose weight. While a person may lose weight initially by removing fat from her diet, there is no way to have a healthy metabolism without consuming healthy fats. Your body must have healthy fats to rebuild the cells. Fat is required to make hormones. A low-fat diet will inevitably lead to a hormone imbalance.

There are two types of fats—real fats and damaged fats. It is important to consume real fats to help maintain a healthy endocrine system.

When choosing which fats to purchase, you will want to note the following on the food labels:

- Damaged fats usually have the words "partially hydrogenated" or "hydrogenated" on the label.
- Damaged fats include margarine and shortening, imitation sour cream, non-dairy creamers, pressurized whipped cream, etc. Contrary to popular belief, margarine is a very unhealthy fat choice.
- Damaged fats also include fats cooked at extremely high heat (such as deep-fried foods).

- Real or "healthful" fats will have the following words: saturated, cold-pressed, pure-pressed, or expeller-pressed mono- or polyunsaturated oils. A few of these include butter, cream, olive oil, grapeseed oil, and canola oil.
- Note that fake fats such as Olestra are man-made and are not healthy for the body.

Recommended Daily Fat Intake:

Your body helps to regulate the amount of healthy fat you eat by secreting a hormone called *colecystokinin*. When you eat fat, the hormone goes to the brain informing it that food has been ingested. If too much of the hormone is released into the blood stream (from eating too much fat), you will become nauseous. (At that point if you continue eating, you will either become more nauseated or vomit.)

Nonstarchy Vegetables

Nonstarchy vegetables provide vitamins, minerals, and fiber for the body.

Vegetables are most healthy when eaten raw. One of the reasons for this is that raw foods are our only source of enzymes, which are needed to properly digest the foods we eat. Heating foods above 105° Fahrenheit kills enzymes. When we do not eat raw foods to provide enzymes for our body, the body becomes the source of the needed enzymes. This, of course, causes an enormous work load on the body. "The energy to digest three meals a day with no enzymes present in the food takes as much energy from the body as an eight-hour work day doing physical labor."[1]

Some nutritional experts suggest that our diet include as much as 50% raw foods each day. There is a lot to be said for the plant foods God has provided for us. It is impossible to improve on God! My pastor of nearly 24 years, Dr. Jack Hyles, used to say, "The closer the food we eat is to the way God made it, the healthier it is for us." (A raw apple is healthier than applesauce which is healthier than apple pie.) The more removed from nature and the more refined food becomes, the less nutrition it provides for our bodies.

Because much of the soil in which the plants are grown is nearly depleted of nutrients, it is best to use organic fruits and vegetables. I realize this is difficult if you live on a limited budget. That is one of the reasons I enjoy the summertime here in Northwest Indiana. I love going to the farmers' market nearly every Saturday morning and stocking up on wonderful fresh produce—much of it organic. I can purchase so much more there for less money than I would spend at the local supermarket, and it is so much fresher!

Since we cannot buy only organic fruits and vegetables, we do two things in our home. First, I purchase an organic cleanser at the health food store called "Dr. Bronner's Sal Suds" to wash all my fruits and vegetables in order to remove pesticides. Second, I take a supplement called Barley

Max. This is actually real food rather than a man-made supplement. It is processed by a company called Hallelujah Acres. (Ordering information is in Appendix C on page 152.) The leaves of very nutrient-rich young organic barley are dried and ground to a powder. Because the process does not heat the leaves above 105° Fahrenheit, the enzymes are left intact, making it a very healthful addition to a regular diet. My pastor's wife takes a nutrient-rich supplement called "blue-green algae" every day. It comes in different forms such as powder and tablets. She uses the tablets as they are easier to manage.

While I usually eat raw vegetables at every meal and snack, I try to eat at least one large salad a day using dark greens such as red leaf, green leaf, and romaine lettuce. (Iceberg lettuce is a man-made hybrid and has little or no fiber or nutritional value.) I like to load up my salad with a great variety of different veggies such as carrots, zucchini, green peppers, red peppers, radishes, chayote squash, yellow squash, tomatoes, cucumbers, cauliflower, broccoli, and more. There are times of the year when some vegetables are not as good (flavorless "pink" tomatoes during the winter months are never on my shopping list, but we eat lots of red, juicy tomatoes during the summer months when I can get them at a very good price at the local farmers' market!) My

> I don't believe exercise is Scriptural. If God had wanted me to touch my toes, He would have put them up higher on my body.

family likes our vegetables cut up in small pieces as it seems to give the salad much more flavor.

I know some people who eat their salads with no dressing, but I have never been able to really enjoy it that way. It is best to use an oil and vinegar dressing for your salad. Just look at the labels to be sure you purchase dressings that are not loaded with sugar and chemicals. Many supermarkets now carry more healthful types of dressings. I have found that some of the Paul Newman dressings are healthful and have great flavor. (I usually use Paul Newman's Olive Oil and Vinegar dressing.)

I have worked to get the cutting and cleaning process of my lettuce down to a science which saves me a lot of time in the long run. In the adjacent box is the procedure I use to keep fresh lettuce in my refrigerator most of the time.

Recommended Daily Nonstarchy Vegetable Intake:
One of the great things about nonstarchy vegetables is that there is no limit to the amount

---

Quick and Easy Preparation for Healthful Salads

• Using a stainless steel knife cut the lettuce very thinly, wash it thoroughly, and then spin it dry in a salad spinner. (I believe everyone who makes salads should own a salad spinner as it so simplifies the process. It helps get the water off of the lettuce, which helps it to last longer.) A stainless steel knife helps keep the lettuce from turning brown as quickly.

• Once the lettuce is cut, washed, and spun, place it in a large glass Pyrex bowl with a plastic lid to store it. The glass bowl seems to keep the lettuce fresher than placing it in plastic.

• Doing several heads of lettuce at a time makes it possible to have lettuce ready for several days to make salads.

---

of nonstarchy veggies you can eat! The other great thing about nonstarchy veggies is that they can be eaten alone. It is best to not eat any of the other food groups alone; they should be eaten with foods from each group. But you can eat nonstarchy veggies anytime apart from any other food groups.

Real Carbohydrates
Carbohydrates are used mainly to fuel the body. There are two types of carbohydrates:
1. The first is *refined carbohydrates* which

The Bakery
A customer in a bakery was observed carefully examining all the rich-looking pastries displayed on trays in the glass cases. When a clerk approached her and asked, "What would you like?" she answered, "I'd like that chocolate-covered, cream-filled doughnut, that jelly-filled doughnut, and that cheese Danish." Then with a sigh she added, "But I'll take an oat bran muffin."

include cookies, cake, candy bars, pop, ice cream, chips, white bread, etc. Refined carbohydrates are made with refined sugars, refined flour, and a number of chemicals. They are empty of any nutritional value and rob you of energy. They actually are considered to be a "toxic chemical" which will be explained in chapter thirteen.

2.   Real or complex carbohydrates include fruits, starchy vegetables, and whole grains.

Recommended Daily Real Carbohydrate Intake:

Carbohydrate intake should be closely monitored. Your body needs real carbohydrates, but, depending on the health of your metabolism, should be limited to the following amounts:

- Consume about 15 to 20 grams of carbohydrates in each of your three meals and at two snack times for a total of about 75 to 100 grams a day.
- As your metabolism begins to heal, increase the amount of carbohydrates at each of your eating times to about 20 to 25 grams.
- Eventually you will increase your intake to about 30 grams at each of your meal times.
- Fruit is a healthy choice for real carbohydrates, but because of the amount of natural sugar in fruit, you should limit fruit intake to three pieces of fruit a day. If you need to lose weight, limit your fruit intake to one piece per day.

- You will want to purchase a carbohydrate counter booklet which indicates the number of carbohydrates in a serving.

When you notice symptoms such as losing weight too quickly (you should not lose more than two pounds a week), waking up during the night from hunger, irritability, or extreme tiredness, you probably are ready to increase your real carbohydrate intake. Please note that during times when you are very active physically, it is important to eat more real carbohydrates since they are mainly used for energy in your body.

At the beginning of this unit explaining the four basic food groups, I mentioned the fact that you should eat three balanced meals a day along with one or two snacks. This is the best way to heal your metabolism. **Never skip meals!** You will never heal your metabolism completely as long as you skip meals or do not get the nutrition you need at each meal.

Eating three balanced meals and two bal-

Bathroom Scales

Two boys were closely examining bathroom scales on display at the department store.

"Have you ever seen one of these before?" one asked.

"Yeah, my mom and dad have one," the other replied.

"What's it for?" asked the first boy.

"I don't know," the second boy answered. "I think you stand on it, and it makes you mad."

anced "snack" meals a day will prevent low blood sugar levels and will also help maintain an even process of rebuilding the cells that are continually being used up.

You will want to refer to Appendix A to help you learn how to plan healthful meals for you and your family. There are many different foods under each of the four food groups, many of which you probably have never tried. You may be surprised to find some new foods that you and your family will enjoy.

An added note to help prepare you for the days ahead as you begin to make changes in your dietary habits: for those ladies who have a very badly damaged metabolism, it is important for you to realize that you may gain some weight initially before you lose weight. *Do not get discouraged. This is part of the healing process to regain a healthy metabolism.* Keep in mind that you are wanting to heal your metabolism so you can lose weight! The weight will come off when you regain a healthy metabolism.

Please Note: I am a very busy wife and mother; I help my husband in the Truck Stop Chapel Ministry; I teach a Sunday school class; I am a name taker at the altar during the invitation; I am a soul winner, and I am involved in other ministries of our church. I also work outside the home. All of that to say, I keep my meals very simple. Eating healthy meals does not have to involve hours and hours of extra work. I do watch for new recipes to keep my menus interest-ing, and I work hard to serve attractive, delicious meals to my family. I do not believe we will stick with something that is complicated. Therefore, I suggest that you keep your menus simple.

Let me give you an example of meals we have eaten in our home recently:

- Grilled chicken breast with fresh sweet corn and a tossed salad with lots of veggies
- Grilled hamburgers with cooked beets and coleslaw
- Eggplant parmigiana with whole grain angel hair pasta and a tossed salad.

I believe you get the idea. Each of these meals brought several thank you's from my family and remarks about how delicious each meal was. Let me encourage you to keep it simple!

Praying for Your Food

Pastor Jack Schaap made some interesting observations in his sermon at First Baptist Church of Hammond, Indiana, on Sunday night, August 20, 2006, regarding the food we eat. This was a very small part of the entire sermon, but it especially arrested my attention since I am writing this book on health. The premise of his teaching was I Timothy 4:4-5 which says, *"For every creature of God is good, and nothing to be refused, if it be received with thanksgiving: **For it is sanctified by the word of God and prayer.**"* Pastor Schaap explained that just as important as the food choices we make is the need to pray over the food we eat. We should ask God to sanctify it and use it to heal, repair, and build up our bodies so we have the strength to do the work He has for us to do. He went on to say that with all the pesticides, chemical additives, lack of proper nutrients, etc. in our food choices, that it is especially important to ask God's intervention in making the food not only safe for us to eat, but also nutritious and filled with the energy our bodies need. What a helpful admonition and explanation of I Timothy 4:4, 5!

As I pondered over his words, I got a new understanding of the importance of praying before meals. I'm afraid that far too many of us pray before meals simply as a habit we learned as young children, and our "prayers" before meals are actually more of a ritual than a prayer. I know that before hearing that sermon, I viewed it more as a time to thank God for the food and His provision. The fact is, I've wondered why we say, "Bless this food to our bodies." What exactly does that mean? I believe it should mean, "Father, sanctify this food and use it to give me the energy and the nutrition I need to make my body healthy."

Pastor Schaap went on to say that possibly some people are sick or in poor health because they fail to ask God to sanctify the food they eat. This reveals to me once again that God is interested in the state of our health. He cares about our health and wants to be involved in our lives. Our health is a spiritual matter as much as it is a physical matter. Therefore, it is vital that we keep God involved.

Hydrating Your Body With Pure Water

Water is an absolute must to regain a healthy metabolism. While it is usually recommended that adults drink eight to ten 8-ounce glasses of pure water each day, many health professionals are now stating that you should drink one half of your body weight in ounces of water a day. For example, a woman who weighs 160 pounds should drink 80 ounces or ten 8-ounce glasses a day. The more you weigh the more fluids your body requires each day. If drinking one half of your body weight in ounces seems too complicated and overwhelming, just start with drinking eight to ten 8-ounce glasses of water a day.

The two best sources for pure water are steam distilled and reverse osmosis. My husband and I purchased a steam distiller from Sears that sits on our counter top in the kitchen. It is much cheaper than purchasing water at the store, and it is

> A man explained to his doctor that he hadn't been feeling well. The doctor examined him, left the room, and came back with three different bottles of pills.
>
> The doctor said, "Take the green pill with a big glass of water when you get up. Take the blue pill with a big glass of water after lunch. Then just before going to bed, take the red pill with another big glass of water."
>
> Startled to be put on so much medicine, the man stammered, "My goodness, Doc, exactly what's my problem?"
>
> The doctor answered, "You're not drinking enough water."

also much easier than "lugging" in bottles from the store.

Why distilled or reverse osmosis? Tap water contains many harmful substances such as chlorine and fluoride. These are toxic (poison) chemicals which cause damage to our bodies. Though many water purifiers do remove some of the harmful substances in tap water, they do not remove them all.

While our bodies can only go without oxygen for a few minutes, water is the second most-needed nutrient in the body. The average person can live quite a few days without food but can only live a few days without water. Why is water such a needed commodity for our bodies?

Our bodies are about 60 percent water; a great amount of water is used by the body each day, and that water needs to be replaced. Water is a cleansing agent in our bodies. When you wash a full load of dirty laundry, what water level setting do you use—small? Absolutely not. You realize that in order for those clothes to get clean they need more than detergent. They need plenty of water to wash the dirt away. So it is for our bodies. Water is a cleansing agent that helps to rid our body of toxins and waste. The body produces waste products in the cells, and water helps wash the waste out of the cells.

Water consumption helps to decrease allergies, arthritic pain, back and neck pain (drinking adequate amounts of water each day over a period of months re-hydrates the disks, causing them to increase in size, thus, reducing your pain and giving you more freedom of movement), and much more. Water also helps to prevent constipation.

Without proper amounts of water your body becomes dehydrated. Some of the symptoms of dehydration include fatigue, bad breath, dry skin, and hunger.

Drinking the appropriate amount of water is pretty much a habit with me now, but when I first attempted to drink eight glasses of water a day I thought I would float away. However, it didn't take long for my body to adjust. I usually drink a 16-ounce glass of water at a time as there's something psychological about four or five glasses of water as opposed to eight or ten!

It is best not to drink a lot of water with your

At the Gym

A lady was self-conscious about going to the gym because she thought the pounds she had put on would make her stand out among the regulars. She chose a treadmill in the corner so she would be inconspicuous.

However, as she exercised, her worst fears came true. At least a dozen people turned to stare at her periodically. She thought it might be her imagination, but then one woman even squinted to get a better look.

Mortified, she stepped off the machine to leave. When she turned around, she realized that the gym's only wall clock had been hanging just inches above her head!

meals as it dilutes your digestive juices and makes digestion more difficult for the body. Also, there is no substitution for pure water. While other drinks contain water (such as coffee, tea, soda, etc.), they do not hydrate and cleanse the body. Because caffeine is a diuretic, you lose more fluid than you drink from beverages that contain caffeine. It actually dehydrates the body. One of the biggest favors you can do your body each day is to drink eight to ten 8-ounce glasses of pure water.

Proper Elimination

There is absolutely no way to maintain a healthy body without proper elimination. In the past I have been told by medical personnel that it is "normal" to have one bowel movement every two to three days. There is no way that can be healthy for the body! A baby has a bowel movement within 30 minutes of each meal. That should be the case for adults also.

Bowel movements eliminate toxic waste from the body. All those cells that are used up, the toxins we ingest—not just those chemicals that we eat in our foods, but also those chemicals we breath and those chemicals that we touch (such as cleaning supplies)—need to be eliminated from the body. It is vital to one's health to have a healthy colon. One cannot have a healthy colon without proper elimination.

The opposite of proper elimination is constipation. There are three main causes of constipation: (1) Poor food choices and not eating enough fiber, (2) Waiting to use the restroom rather than eliminating the waste immediately, and (3) Not drinking enough water.

Of course, the obvious fixes for those three causes include:

1. Eating plenty of fiber-rich foods (plant foods) especially nonstarchy vegetables

2. Use the restroom immediately when the urge comes

3. Drink eight to ten 8-ounce glasses of pure water a day. Waste products cannot move efficiently through 30 feet of intestines without adequate amounts of water!

4. Take some type of natural fiber which is available at health food stores. A physician once said to me, "Short of dynamite, take something so you have at least one bowel movement daily." Laxatives are the number-one selling over-the-counter drugs in America. Making the four changes I suggested in this paragraph would greatly reduce the need for laxatives (which are usually made with toxic chemicals) and would greatly improve the health of those using the laxatives!

It is disgusting to realize that when waste cannot get out of your system due to constipation, the toxins are reabsorbed into the body! There is a large body of water in the Holy Land that takes in and takes in and takes in, but there are no outlets releasing water. It is called the Dead Sea. That is a pretty good indication of what happens to our bodies when we continually take in food without proper elimination.

Eating a balanced diet, drinking plenty of pure water, and proper elimination are the first steps you should take in attempting to heal your metabolism. It will not take you long to feel some of the benefits of making the necessary changes in your lifestyle habits.

Step One Principles

- Eat three meals each day and one to two snack "meals" each consisting of food from each of the four basic food groups.
- Drink at least eight to ten 8-ounce glasses of pure water each day.
- Eliminate waste and toxins from your body each day with regular bowel movements.

The Benefits of Health Food

An 85-year-old couple, having been married almost 60 years, died in a car crash. They had been in good health the last ten years mainly due to her interest in health food and exercise.

When they reached the pearly gates, St. Peter took them to their mansion which was decked out with a beautiful kitchen, master bath suite, and a Jacuzzi. As they "oohed and aahed," the man asked Peter how much all this was going to cost. "It's free," Peter replied. "This is Heaven." Next they went out back to survey the championship golf course that was connected to their home. They would have golfing privileges every day, and each week the course changed to a new one representing the great golf courses on earth.

The old man asked, "What are the green fees?"

Peter's reply, "This is Heaven; you play for free."

Next they went to the clubhouse and saw the lavish buffet lunch with all types of delicious cuisines. "How much does it cost to eat?" asked the old man.

"Don't you understand yet? This is Heaven; it is free!" Peter replied with some exasperation.

"Well, where are the low-fat and low-cholesterol tables?" the old man asked timidly.

Peter lectured, "That's the best part…you can eat as much as you like of whatever you like, and you never get fat, and you never get sick. This is Heaven."

With that the old man went into a fit of anger, throwing down his hat and stomping on it, and shrieking wildly. Peter and his wife both tried to calm him down, asking him what was wrong. The old man looked at his wife and said, "This is all your fault. If it weren't for your blasted bran muffins, I could have been here ten years ago!"

Proper Sleep and Stress Management

The second step toward healing your metabolism is proper sleep and stress management. For the most part, this is a matter of structuring your life and your thinking.

Everyone experiences two types of stress which must be managed: physical and emotional. The first stress we experience is physical stress. Our bodies are in a constant state of using up and rebuilding cells. How efficiently our bodies go through that process indicates the health of our metabolism. The using up and rebuilding of all of our biochemicals takes its toll (a stress, if you will) on our bodies, thus requiring energy. Therefore, our bodies require rest (i.e. **sleep**)! The second stress we experience is emotional stress. This includes everything from small irritations or frustrations such as losing your car keys to "big ticket items" like a death in the family, a wayward child, or a divorce.

Proper Sleep

Not getting enough sleep prevents the body from recovering from the physical stress it endures each day and contributes to a damaged metabolism. To keep the using-up side of your metabolism in balance with the replacement side of your metabolism, you must have adequate sleep. *There is no substitute for sleep.*

Sleep also gives your body the rest it needs to be able to properly deal with the *emotional stress* you face each day. The great football coach Vince Lombardi once said, "Fatigue makes cowards of us all." Depriving our bodies of sleep affects our ability to face struggles and crises in our lives.

Your body can only heal when you are sleeping. When you are awake and active, your body is expending energy. Your body's healing hormones are released when you are sleeping so it can repair and regenerate itself. Your body gets its best rest by going to bed as soon as possible after the sun goes down. The hours you sleep before midnight are twice as effective for rebuilding and restoring than those after midnight.[1]

David L. Katz, M.D., is the director of the Prevention Research Center at Yale University School of Medicine. He says regarding the correlation of sleep and obesity, "Sleep is directly related to weight loss in that if you don't get enough of it, it could cause you to gain weight or have trouble losing it. Here's why: Studies show that regularly getting less than seven hours of sleep a night lowers the appetite-suppressing hormone leptin and raises the appetite-promoting hormone ghrelin. If you get enough sleep, not only do your hormones stay balanced, but your basal (resting) metabolism can go to work burning calories straight through the night. And getting enough sleep also makes it easier to cope with the daily stresses that could trigger overeating."[2]

Live by schedule. It is best for your body to be on a regular schedule, not only for sleeping but for every area of your life. The human body responds to and thrives on routine. Going to bed at the same time, getting up at the same time, eating meals at the same time, and carrying out other responsibilities of life at the same time each day enhances the body's ability to heal. The structured

life is an ally to a healthy body and will accelerate the healing process. I Corinthians 14:40 says, *"Let all things be done decently and in order."* Ecclesiastes 3:1-8 lists different times for doing things. *"To every thing there is a season, and a time to every purpose under the heaven: A time to be born, and a time to die; a time to plant, and a time to pluck up that which is planted; A time to kill, and a time to heal; a time to break down, and a time to build up; A time to weep, and a time to laugh; a time to mourn, and a time to dance; A time to cast away stones, and a time to gather stones together; a time to embrace, and a time to refrain from embracing; A time to get, and a time to lose; a time to keep, and a time to cast away; A time to rend, and a time to sew; a time to keep silence, and a time to speak; A time to love, and a time to hate; a time of war, and a time of peace."*

God loves schedule and routine. We are made in His image. The Bible clearly teaches that He wants the same of us. He knows we'll be healthier, happier, and more productive because of it.

In a Sunday evening sermon concerning health, especially women's health, my pastor admonished us to get seven to eight hours of sleep a night. My pastor is the very busy pastor of the great First Baptist Church of Hammond, Indiana, a many-faceted megachurch, but he realizes the importance of proper sleep. In order for your biochemicals to properly rebuild, you should get seven to eight hours of *uninterrupted* sleep a night. Studies show that the majority of women struggling with weight control and not feeling

Tofu Receipes

A well-dressed man approached a woman at a health food store and in a clipped British accent asked her exactly what she did with the tofu in her basket.

She answered, "Normally, I put it in the refrigerator, look at it for several weeks, and then throw it away."

The man replied, "That's exactly what my wife does with it. I was hoping you had a better recipe."

well are sleep deprived; sleep deprivation leads to a damaged metabolism. The studies done on sleep indicate that the majority of obese women do not get proper sleep.

As Christians it is easy to believe that we are doing a good thing to deprive ourselves of sleep in order to do a work for God. That is a lie of the Devil. Though there are times we need to get less sleep to do an eternal work (such as conferences, vacation Bible school, etc.) those should be exceptions to the rule rather than the regular routine of life. The Devil is a "big picture" guy. He has patience. He can wait a few years for one of his lies to bring the desired results. Getting the proper rest is a very spiritual decision.

My church, First Baptist Church of Hammond, Indiana, hosts three major conferences each year: Pastors' School the third week in March, Youth Conference in July, and the Christian Womanhood Spectacular International Ladies' Conference the third week of October. My family is very involved in each of these conferences and has a number of responsibilities that involve getting up and being at the church early in the morning and getting home quite late each evening. We go into each of these conferences realizing that we will be somewhat sleep-deprived at the end of the week. Therefore, we make plans to get extra rest the week following each conference.

There are other similar situations, such as a the arrival of a new baby. A mother of a newborn infant does not have the liberty to say, "I'm going to close the baby's door and my door so I don't hear crying in the night. I need my eight hours of sleep!" It just doesn't work that way. However, some plans should be made for the new mother to get the rest she needs to be able to function properly. When our daughter Carissa was born, my husband helped me to set up some guidelines for me to get rest.

• We planned that I would take a nap when Carissa was sleeping. Sometimes I felt like I needed to use that time to get things done, but I quickly realized that taking a much-needed nap helped me to be more efficient and productive than if I tried to work when I needed that nap.

• I let people help me when they offered. Some were family members who came from out of town for even as briefly as a day or just overnight. They did some cleaning for me, watched Carissa so I could go grocery shopping or run errands, etc. I also had friends and church members cook meals for me. All of those things enabled me to get some extra rest. Our pride sometimes gets in the way, so we don't want to let others help us. Accept the help so you can get your rest!

It is especially important that a person get extra

> **Eat Your Vegetables!**
> Chocolate is derived from cacao beans. Beans are a vegetable. Sugar is derived from either sugar CANE or sugar BEETS. Both are plants, which places them in the vegetable category. Thus, chocolate is a vegetable.

> **Sales Rep to Physician:** Our new synthetic fat substitute is made entirely from wool. With our product, dieters will shrink when they get wet!

rest during times of great emotional stress. I was out of town when I received word that a sweet couple in our church had lost their young infant. I was not going to be able to go to the funeral, so I decided to call and let the mother know that I was thinking of her and praying for her and her family. When her husband answered the phone, I told him who I was and asked if I could speak with his wife for a few minutes. He kindly told me that she was taking a nap. I was thrilled and asked him not to wake her. This was a very wise woman who realized (or possibly her husband realized) that she needed extra rest during this time of tremendous emotional stress on her body.

Guidelines for Proper Sleep:

1. **Go to bed early enough to give yourself time to relax and fall asleep.** For example, if you need to get up at 6:00 a.m., you should be asleep by 10:00 p.m. If it takes you an hour to fall asleep, go to bed at 9:00 p.m.

If you are suffering from adrenal burnout, it is important to be in bed and asleep before your "second wind" hits about 11:00 p.m. Staying up late will further exhaust your adrenals.

2. **Resist the urge to get back out of bed when you don't fall asleep immediately.** Stay in bed. When I can't get to sleep, I am tempted to get back out of bed and accomplish things around the house. This is neither restful to my husband nor to me. It simply complicates the problem.

3. **Claim Psalm 127:2, "…he [the LORD] giveth his beloved sleep…."** I pray and say, "Lord, You know that I need sleep in order to heal my metabolism and have the strength I need to function properly tomorrow. I trust You to keep Your Word promising that You give Your beloved sleep." Then I begin quoting that verse or another Bible passage (usually one I am working on memorizing at that time) slowly over and over in my mind until I fall asleep.

4. **Try to drink most of your liquids earlier in the day so you don't have to get up in the night to use the restroom.**

5. **If necessary, take natural sleep-aid supplements available at health food stores.** I do not encourage the use of drugs because they are toxic chemicals to your body and further damage your metabolism. Though melatonin is often recommended, inositol is considered a better sleep aid to use. (Melatonin can have adverse effects on your metabolism.)

6. **If you can't get eight hours of sleep with your schedule, get seven.** Eight hours is preferable, but sometimes our schedules do not permit that amount of time. However, every night you are able to get those eight hours of sleep, you are helping your metabolism to heal.

7. Realize you will not heal your metabolism overnight. It took years to wear your body down. You may find as you start getting extra sleep, you want even more. That is normal. If you can have nights periodically where you get ten or twelve hours of sleep, do so.

I can testify to the fact that if your body is sleep deprived, you will probably need some of those longer nights. I did. But I am finding that as I get good, consistent sleep, I am now waking up much more refreshed…and waking up before the alarm clock! It's a wonderful feeling to wake up feeling rested and able to get out of bed ready to face the day.

Sometimes I have ladies tell me they feel lazy if they get that much sleep. Proverbs 6:9–11 says, *"How long wilt thou sleep, O sluggard? when wilt thou arise out of thy sleep? Yet a little sleep, a little slumber, a little folding of the hands to sleep: So shall thy poverty come as one that travelleth, and thy want as an armed man."* There are lazy people who, because of a lack of character, sleep way more than they need to sleep. They laze around during the day, don't live by schedule, and accomplish very little in life.

This is not the type of extra sleep I am talking about. Probably if you are reading this book and seeking answers to your health problems, you are not a lazy person. Now, there is no doubt that a damaged metabolism and hormonal imbalances cause fatigue. It is not uncommon for obese people to feel tired all the time and want to sleep a lot. That is why it is so important to make changes in one's eating habits first and foremost. Getting extra sleep without changing other lifestyle choices that cause a damaged metabolism (especially poor nutrition) will not be nearly as effective in healing your body.

It is not laziness to get the sleep our bodies need (including that initial extra amount of sleep needed in our first stage of healing). God designed our bodies to need rest. It is important to note as you read the Gospels, that Jesus got tired, and when He did, He rested. *(What a way to be like Jesus!)*

Handling Emotional Stress Scripturally

Stress is defined as "the psychological strain you encounter on a day-to-day basis." It would be ideal to be able to get rid of all stress, but that will not happen until we get to Heaven. Every person in the world deals with emotional stress—including children and babies (from trying to communicate that they are hungry or need a dia-

A young lady was visiting a psychiatrist, hoping to cure her eating and sleeping disorder. "Every thought I have turns to my mother," she told the psychiatrist. "As soon as I fall asleep and begin to dream, everyone in my dream turns into my mother. I wake up so upset that all I can do is go downstairs and eat a piece of toast."

The psychiatrist replied, "What, just one piece of toast for a big girl like you?"

per change to mastering new milestones such as rolling over, sitting up, crawling, walking, etc.)

When we are in stressful situations, our bodies secrete a hormone called cortisol to help us cope. When a person faces extreme stress over an extended period of time, her body continues to secrete cortisol. When this happens, she depletes her body of cortisol which contributes to a hormonal imbalance in the body (and, of course, an unhealthy metabolism). Adrenal gland burnout is

Women's Remarks for High Stress Days

1. Well, this day was a total waste of make-up.
2. I'm not crazy; I've just been in a very bad mood for over 30 years.
3. Allow me to introduce myselves.
4. Sarcasm is just one more service we offer.
5. Whatever kind of look you were going for, you missed.
6. I'm trying to imagine you with a personality.
7. Stress is when you wake up screaming and you realize you weren't asleep.
8. I can't remember if I'm the good twin or the evil one.
9. Can I trade this job for what's behind door #2?
10. Nice perfume. Must you marinate in it?
11. Is it time for your medication or mine?
12. How do I set a laser printer to stun?
13. I'm not tense, just terribly, terribly alert.

a common problem among women. Therefore, it is vital that we take the necessary steps to properly deal with emotional stress in our lives. Our health depends on it!

I have come to the conclusion that often the amount of stress our bodies experience does not have as much to do with the source of the stress as it does with our response to the stress. I have seen people go through unbelievable valleys and remain pretty steady while others go ballistic and worry for days that their child is going to get terribly sick or even die because he did something like put his hand in the toilet. What makes the difference? It has a lot to do with our thinking and how we allow or discipline our minds to respond to stressful situations.

I think of Marlene Evans (the founder of Christian Womanhood) who fought cancer for almost 20 years—first breast cancer and then ovarian. She faced a lot of negative news, especially being told that she had ovarian cancer, stage IV and that she had probably 18 months to 2½ years to live. She knew that meant more chemotherapy treatments, surgery, and the like, but she kept a great attitude and lived her life influencing others for eternity until her body succumbed to the cancer. I believe her response to emotional stress was Scriptural, which helped her prolong her life.

Following are principles that will help you face emotional stresses in a Scriptural manner and which will help you heal a damaged metabolism.

Walk With God!

John 15:5b says, " *...for without me ye can do nothing.*" We cannot deal with stress in a Biblical manner if we are not daily walking with God in prayer, Bible reading, Bible memorization, praise, and so forth.

I had a wonderful blessing at work one day. A dear lady had purchased the book I wrote entitled *Losing Weight–Gaining Control,* a 26-week Bible study on weight control, which also includes basic principles to regaining a healthy metabolism. This lady wrote to tell me that though she is regaining her health and had lost nine pounds to date, the greatest blessing is that the book helped her get in the habit of reading her Bible every day. I could not have been more thrilled because the first step toward finding solutions to any problem is walking with God! The answers we need will be found in the Bible and on our knees in prayer.

Do you walk with God on a daily basis? If you do, wonderful! If you do not have a daily walk with God, begin today! If you don't, it is probably because you don't have a plan. There are many resources available; let me suggest two. The senior editor of *Christian Womanhood*, Mrs. Cindy Schaap, has a monthly planner entitled, *Living on the Bright Side Journal.* The second suggested Bible and prayer journal is *Ready for the Day!* by Loretta Walker. Both of these include Bible reading plans and prayer schedules, and both are available through Christian Womanhood.

Walking with God gives us a *"peace...which passeth all understanding."* There's no better time than today to begin your walk with God and to begin your journey of dealing with stress in a practical, Biblical way.

Praise God

To most Christians, Romans chapter one is a familiar passage which explains the progression people take toward wickedness, ultimately ending in destruction. Verse 21 says, *"Because that, when they knew God, they glorified him not as God, neither were thankful...."* These people committed a number of offenses, but the first two God mentioned were not worshipping Him and being unthankful. They did not praise God. Dr. Jack Schaap, says, "Praise is one of the greatest weapons we have against temptation." Praising God helps us live the victorious Christian life.

Most Christians have a fair amount of negative in their lives. I believe this is especially true of those who are trying to live the Spirit-filled life and a life of obedience to God because the Devil wants to defeat them. However, no matter how negative our circumstances seem or how much goes wrong in our lives, we are commanded to praise God. First Thessalonians 5:16 and 18 say, *"Rejoice evermore.... In every thing give thanks: for this is the will of God in*

> **Patient to Dietician:**
> "If a vegetarian diet is good for losing weight, how come they use grain to fatten pigs and cows?"

Christ Jesus concerning you." Philippians 4:4 says, *"Rejoice in the Lord alway: and again I say, Rejoice."*

One of the key reasons praise and rejoicing are such an important part of a victorious life is that our thought processes have so much to do with how we act. That which we speak to ourselves in our minds is that which we act out in our lives. How and what I think also determines how I feel. Negative feelings lead to depression, which, of course, contributes to a damaged metabolism.

Do you have a difficult time thinking of things for which to praise God? We shouldn't for He has done so much for us, but if negative thoughts have reigned in our lives (especially negative thoughts about ourselves and our situations), it can sometimes be difficult to get started.

God gives us many reasons for which to praise Him, but one of my favorite passages to turn to when I seem to be losing my praise is Psalm 103. In fact, it is such a praise chapter I would encourage you to memorize it. We are commanded in verse two of that chapter, *"Bless the LORD, O my soul, and forget not all his benefits."* Psalm 68:19 says, *"Blessed be the LORD, who daily loadeth us with benefits, even the God of our salvation. Selah."*

What are some of these benefits God loads upon us daily? I will not go through the entire chapter, but the following are just a few of the benefits listed in Psalm 103:

Verse 3 — He forgives our iniquities, and He heals us.

Verse 4 — He redeems us, and He crowns us (or encircles us for protection) with lovingkindness and tender mercies.

Verse 5 — He satisfies our mouth with good things.

Verse 8 — He is merciful and gracious, and He is plenteous in mercy.

Wow! Get the idea? We have a great God! When we are thinking and talking about how good He is to us, all that He has done for us, and all that He continues to do for us, we cannot, at the same time, be thinking negative, destructive thoughts which lead to defeat in our lives and contribute to emotional stress and a damaged metabolism.

Chemical Analysis of Human Elements

Element name: WOMAN

Symbol: WO

Atomic weight: *"Don't even go there."*

Physical properties: Generally round in form. Boils at nothing and may freeze at any time. Melts whenever treated properly. Very bitter if not used well.

Chemical properties: Very active. Highly unstable. Possesses strong affinity to gold, silver, platinum, and precious gemstones. Violent when left alone. Able to absorb great amounts of exotic food. Turns slightly green when placed next to a better specimen.

Usage: Highly ornamental. An extremely good catalyst for dispersion of wealth. Probably the most powerful income reducing agent known.

Caution: Highly explosive in inexperienced hands.

It seems that when we are not feeling well, negative thoughts and emotions come so much more easily. In May of 2004 I had neck surgery. One morning shortly after surgery I awoke with the feeling that there were dark clouds all around me. Everything seemed so black. I could almost feel waves of negative thoughts and emotions rolling toward me as if to drown me. I immediately started praising God, but it was as if an oppressive spirit was around me. I then began praising God out loud and singing praise songs. I finally said aloud, "Devil, you are not welcome here. Get out!" I continued praising God, and peace came. (I was on pain medication, and I realize pain-relieving drugs, especially narcotics, can also greatly affect your spirit. It was sweet to me that God is more powerful than the Devil and the side effects of pain medication!)

I believe that had I given in to those negative emotions and thoughts and allowed them to have free reign in my life that morning, I would have lived a day of defeat and misery. Praise is a wonderful enabler God has given us to help us live the victorious Christian life. Praise will enable us to be more victorious in our struggle and will help us heal our metabolism. Let's use it!

Exercise Mind Control

Earlier in this chapter I mentioned Marlene Evans as a great example of dealing with stress in a Scriptural

I don't suffer from anxiety. I enjoy every minute of it.

manner. The key? One of the greatest attributes of Mrs. Evans was that she had learned the Scriptural concept of controlling her thought life. She even gave a speech at one of the Christian Womanhood Spectaculars entitled, "Mind Control."

Mrs. Evans decided what thoughts she was going to allow into her mind. I believe that one of the big reasons why she lived for more than seven years after her diagnosis rather than the short time predicted was that she decided not to place additional stress on her body with negative thinking.

Now, she did not put her head in the sand and pretend she didn't have cancer. She did not live in denial. Rather, she asked questions to find out the facts, she asked questions and researched what steps she could take to best fight her cancer (looking into and using both traditional and alternative methods of treatment), and she worked to institute those ideas. Then she kept her mind on things other than her cancer.

She had to fight depression as much or more than anyone. She had to fight dwelling on her negative cancer diagnosis as much as anyone. The difference was that she decided not to give a lot of attention to the negative. I learned a wonderful principle for mind control from Mrs. Evans through my good friend Carol Tudor.

Carol was my dormitory supervisor for one year at Hyles-Anderson College. We had dorm devotions several nights a week. On one particular night she taught on mind control. She used a chair to symbolize the mind. She had a girl sit on the chair representing a negative thought. She said that oftentimes when we are convicted of thinking negative thoughts, we say to ourselves, "I shouldn't be thinking about this," and try to quit thinking that thought. However, thinking about trying to get rid of the negative thinking does not get rid of the negative thinking. We are still dwelling on it as we think, "I shouldn't be thinking about this." Carol had the young lady (representing the negative thought) get back on the chair. She then chose another young lady to represent a good or positive thought (a Philippians 4:8 thought—*"Finally, brethren, whatsoever things are true, whatsoever things are honest, whatsoever things are just, whatsoever things are pure, whatsoever things are lovely, whatsoever things are of good report; if there be any virtue, and if there be any praise, think on these things."*) When the negative thought came, she had the young lady representing a good thought move onto the chair, pushing the other young lady (representing a negative or bad thought) off of the chair. It is the principle of "replacement." Rather than trying to get rid of the negative thought, simply pull in a positive thought which will automatically force the negative or sinful thought out of your mind. It's a rather simple principle really. It just takes the discipline not to allow the negative to dwell in your mind—and to pull the right thoughts in to replace them.

Our thought life determines our attitude and the way we handle stress. Let me give you an example. When something negative happens, we have two choices. First, we can get upset at God and complain to Him and to anyone else who will listen as to how unfair life is. We can choose to allow very negative thoughts to rule our minds and live in depression. All of this causes excessive stress on our bodies and further damages our metabolism.

The second choice is to immediately thank God for the trial and find ways to praise Him. I'm not suggesting you "high-five" everyone you come in contact with over your emotional stress. But realizing that God is in control and has allowed the negative situation will help you get your bearings and be able to face the trial in a much more calm and peaceful way. The key is controlling your thought life.

I have learned a wonderful phrase from Mrs. Cindy Schaap regarding mind control. Though she is the wife of the pastor of a very large church, she is not exempt from the temptation to think negative, critical, or wrong thoughts. She has given her testimony a number of times as to how, as a young college student, she laughed when she heard the principle of mind control taught. She thought it was impossible to control one's thought life. However, she has learned that it is very possible since it is a command of God. When she is tempted to think negative, critical, bitter, or any other kind

> **Waitress to Customer:**
> The diet special is a tiny green salad without dressing, a large glass of ice water, and two desserts.

of wrong thoughts, she says to herself, "Whoa! I'm not goin' there!" and refuses to allow her mind to think on the wrong thoughts. That statement has become a regular part of my response to wrong thinking, "Whoa, I'm not goin' there!" Just refuse to let your mind go wild thinking negative, hurtful, destructive thoughts.

Thank God for Everything

Stress is one of those subtle, quiet enemies to good health that wreaks havoc on our bodies while we obliviously continue our unhealthy lifestyle of not dealing with our stress in a Biblical manner. None of us can keep stress from our lives, but we can determine the way in which we handle the stresses. Stress is very much about perception and response.

Watch a young child throw a temper tantrum over not getting his way—a big stress item to a toddler. I was in a store recently when a toddler's mother told him "No."

He immediately threw himself onto the floor and began kicking and screaming. That boy had a lot of stress in his life over being told "No."

Now you and I think it's ridiculous to throw ourselves on the floor to kick and scream over a small, inexpensive toy or a piece of candy. Yet adults by the thousands, yes, even Christian adults, throw temper tantrums of their own sort over negatives that come into their lives. When events or hurts come into our lives, we immediately get "bent out of shape" and start "yelling" at God and telling Him how unfair and unkind He is to allow this hurt. Simply put, we don't let God be God.

• James 1:2—"*My brethren, **count it all joy** when ye fall into divers temptations.*" That word *temptations* means "testing." We are commanded to count it all joy when tests and trials (stresses!) come our way. Why? Let's read verses three and four of James chapter one—"*Knowing this, that the trying of your faith worketh patience. But let patience have her perfect work, that ye may be perfect and*

Diets and Donuts

A devout woman who was very overweight decided to go on a diet. One of her main problems with eating was that she would stop for donuts every morning on the way to work. To make things easier for herself, she changed her route to work to avoid the temptation of stopping.

As the weeks went by, she started losing a lot of weight and was receiving compliments from her friends and co-workers.

Then, one morning without thinking, she accidentally turned on the road which would take her by the donut shop. At first she was going to turn around, but then she thought to herself, "Maybe the Lord is rewarding me for my efforts." So, she said a short prayer telling the Lord that if this was His true intention (for her to go to the donut shop) that He would let there be an open parking place directly in front of the shop. Sure enough, on the eighth time around the block there was an open spot right in front of the bakery!

entire, wanting nothing."

In order for us to become mature, complete Christians, God knows that we need trials and testings in our lives. We do not have a mean God Who sits in the Heavenlies trying to figure out how complicated and unnerving He can make our lives each day. He does, however, continue to allow testings, frustrations, and trials in our lives to help us grow and reach our potential.

• I Thessalonians 5:18—*"In every thing give thanks: for this is the will of God in Christ Jesus concerning you."* I've heard sermons explaining this verse in two ways. The first is that it is the will of God for you to rejoice in everything that comes your way. The second is that whatever comes your way is the will of God and allowed by Him. I believe both are correct. We are to thank God for everything He allows.

Now, does that mean when the doctor tells you that you have cancer you say, "Wahoo! I've got cancer! Not only that, but my husband has cancer, my child has cancer; and even my dog has cancer! We're just one big happy cancer family! Wahoo! Wahoo! Wahoo!" Absolutely not.

When the trials come, God understands our tears, our disappointment, and our hurting heart. Psalm 56:8 indicates God keeps our tears in a bottle. Our tears are precious to Him. God expects us to grieve and hurt, but through the grief and hurt we should

> Remember, "STRESSED" spelled backward is "DESSERTS."

get to God and say something like, "Father, you know I would not have chosen this hurt in my life, but I trust You. You know what I need in my life to become all you want me to be. I'm asking for Your help to go through this trial in a way that will bring glory and honor to Your name. I'm asking that whatever eternal purpose You have for allowing this hurt will be fulfilled."

To thank God for the stress that comes into your life means realizing that God allowed this hurt for a purpose. We serve an "on purpose" God Who has a goal to accomplish in everything He does. All that He does is for an eternal good. We may not even see the eternal good in our lifetime, but God knows what He is doing. Romans 8:28 says, *"And we know that all things work together for good to them that love God, to them who are the called according to his purpose."* Our pastor says in explanation of this verse, "When someone succeeds without suffering, it is because someone somewhere suffered without succeeding."

We don't understand the mysteries of God and the ways He works. I can only tell you that when He allows struggles, hurts, and disappointments in your life, He does it for good. His plan is not for you to resist that hurt to the detriment of your health.

When the hurts come, rather than allowing yourself to get upset, mad at God, and question why He would let such a trial in your life, take a deep breath, relax, and thank Him for allowing this in your life. Then ask Him for the grace to go through the trial in a way that will glorify Him and fulfill His eternal purpose.

It is normal that you have tears in difficult times. Psalm 142:1 says that David cried to God. That word *cried* in that passage indicates that he continually cried. He did not just cry to God once. He was under tremendous stress as King Saul was after him to kill him, so he cried repeatedly to God on a consistent basis. God expects your tears through the trials, but He also wants you to have joy through the tears.

Negative stress handled in a negative way brings tremendous stress to your body affecting the health and well-being of your body. Negative stress will come, but prepare yourself to *"count it all joy"* and to *"give thanks"* to God for all that He allows to come your way.

Laugh a Lot

Proverbs 17:22 says, " *A merry heart doeth good like a medicine: but a broken spirit drieth the bones.* " Laughter is a gift from God which contributes to a healthy body. "On average, children laugh 400 times a day; adults laugh only 25. Laughter decreases blood pressure, boosts the immune system, and more. Laughter does good like a medicine."[3]

Usually the times we find it most difficult to laugh are times we need to laugh the most. When I don't feel well, not much seems funny or humorous. Praise the

> I'm in shape. Round is a shape.

Lord I have a husband who has a great sense of humor! He provides a lot of laughter for me when I seem to need it the most. My pastor's wife says that she has a friend who is hysterically funny, and when she really needs to laugh, she calls that friend. If you are in such a difficult situation that you find it hard to laugh or have fun, let me give you some thoughts from Marlene Evans' book *Comfort for Hurting Hearts.* You would benefit from reading the entire chapter she has written on "Jesus Our Fun."

- Watch kids.
- Read funny stories and jokes.
- Make light of the heavy.
- Seek to be with fun people.
- Turn frustrations into jokes.
- Exaggerate everyday happenings.
- Laugh at yourself.
- Check that which makes people laugh.

Everyone needs to laugh, but if you have a damaged metabolism, be sure that laughing is a regularly scheduled event in your life. Laughing will help your body to heal. The word *merry* in Proverbs 17:22 gives the idea of deep, hearty laughter. In no way does it seem to indicate a little smirk or small chuckle. A merry heart is one that displays a joyful, excited spirit. Years ago I had a friend who would barely smirk when people would say some of the funniest things. One day another friend said, "Don't you think things are funny?"

My friend was shocked and said, "Yes, I just laugh on the inside."

My other friend quickly responded, "Why don't you notify your face and the rest of the world that you think things are funny." This was a new thought to that friend. From that day until this, she laughs a hearty laugh when things are humorous. What a teachable spirit she had. Whether she realized it or not, she was helping to build her immune system and bringing health to her body! Laugh! Laugh! Laugh!

Refuse to be Easily Offended

Psalm 119: 165 says, *"Great peace have they which love thy law: and nothing shall offend them."* If you are a person who is easily offended, I can guarantee that your hurt feelings add tremendous emotional stress to your life. I was a person who was quite easily offended. While some people are blatant about displaying their offended spirit, I think I was somewhat of a "closet" offendee (if there is such a word!). I nursed my hurt feelings privately which led to a depressed spirit. I also was cool in my treatment of those who offended me.

When I moved to Indiana in 1977 to attend Hyles-Anderson College, I asked Carol Frye Tudor how to get over being easily offended. What a favor she did me that day when she quoted Psalm 119:165. I thought that her solution sounded too simple (I have since learned that when I tell myself that a solution someone gives me is "too simple," the problem is not

> *"I've tried relaxing, but I feel more comfortable tense."*

that it's too simple; the problem is that my pride is not wanting to obey the Bible.)

The next time I was offended happened to be by Carol and my friend Kris who is now my sister-in-law! They went shopping and did not ask me to go along! I got hurt and went to my dorm room, got my nightgown on, and went to bed. It was about 6:00 in the evening! Looking back I remind myself of Ahab when Naboth would not sell Ahab his vineyard! I laid down and allowed my mind to go wild thinking things like, "I am not going to speak to them until they apologize," and other ridiculous thoughts. After a few minutes the Holy Spirit reminded me of Carol's instruction just a few days prior. I argued in my mind, "Well, I have a right to be offended this time; they mistreated me."

The Holy Spirit won, I got out of bed, and I looked up the verse. (I couldn't remember the verse number, but I remembered the essence of the verse, so I had to read all the way to 165 to find it. God knew I needed all the Scripture I could get!) I began quoting the verse, but as soon as I quoted it, my mind would go back to those negative thoughts. I started quoting it faster and faster so I would not have time to think the negative thoughts. After quoting the verse about 75 to 100 times, I suddenly had peace. It was at that point that I realized Carol and Kris had done absolutely nothing wrong. After all, there is nowhere in the Bible that says, "Thou shalt always include every friend in your invitation to go to the mall!" or any verse close to that! My offense came because I was selfish, and my selfishness caused me to be out of perspective.

That was a turning point for me. I do not believe anyone would say now that I am characterized by being easily offended. Because I am human, I, of course, do sometimes get offended, but it is no longer a "way of life" for me, and I am more quickly able to work though the hurt feelings and go on with life. Hanging on to hurts causes us to have to carry a lot of excess baggage with us everywhere we go.

Being offended is a sin. It is one of the works of the flesh (which is a doorway for unclean spirits to enter our lives) listed in Galatians chapter five. Verse 20 uses the word *emulations* which simply means "overly sensitive." Claim Psalm 119:165 to get victory over being easily offended. Claim Psalm 119:165 to help prevent unnecessary emotional stress from attacking your metabolism!

Where are you on the emotional stress scale? If you live "stressed out" most of the time, you need to consider making changes to help heal your body. There is no doubt that emotional stress takes its toll on your body, but your attitude and response to the stress that comes your way is a key to protecting your metabolism.

When Stress Makes You Want to Eat!

While some women say, "I'm so upset I just can't eat,"

> A balanced diet is a cookie in each hand.

when they face emotional stress, many of us automatically reach for food. It doesn't even seem to matter what food we eat, .We eat whatever is available as an automatic response to emotional stress.

Several times a year I travel out of town to speak at ladies' meetings. On one particular occasion, I had just returned home from Marysville, Washington. When I walked into the kitchen, I noticed a mixing bowl filled with white powder and melted butter, slightly mixed together. I questioned my husband, and he said, "While Carissa [our teenage daughter] was working on her term paper, I told her I would make chocolate chip cookies." Tom, who has a great sense of humor, then dramatically opened the cupboard doors, pointed to my canisters neatly lined up in a row, and asked dryly, "What do these containers say?"

As I answered, "Flour, flour...." I immediately realized he had used confectioner's sugar instead of flour. My husband thought if the canister said "flour" on the outside, surely that's what was inside, but that wasn't so in my cupboards! (For the well-being of all involved, I have since fixed this discrepancy that I had failed to care for when I purchased some new canisters and started putting confectioner's sugar into the old flour container!)

So it is when we think we are hungry. Certain stimuli trigger my feelings to think I'm hungry. I find myself eating ravenously when in reality I'm not hungry at all.

That same year, a week before Pastors' School at First Baptist Church of Hammond, Christian

Womanhood was asked to conduct the afternoon ladies' sessions in addition to its regular duties at Pastors' School. I was busy and feeling a little stressed as I was trying to meet typesetting and printing deadlines. I had to take a layout to the printer. It was a little past my regular lunchtime, so on my way I stopped at Zel's Drive Thru and ordered a roast beef sandwich and fries. (I reasoned, "I can eat the fries because I'm drinking water and not eating the bread!") I ate that lunch, dropped off the layout, and then stopped at home to change clothes before driving to the mall to get our group picture taken for the Christian Womanhood Spectacular ad. I found myself searching for food and grabbing a handful of coconut (left over from the chocolate chip cookies my husband had made while I was gone!)

I suddenly stopped as I realized my eating was out of control. As I questioned why I was eating, I came to the conclusion that I was eating because I was stressed. (I'm sorry, but I do not relate to women who say, "I'm too nervous [or too busy] to eat.") I knew I had to do something right then, or I would be out of control the rest of the day. I went to my computer and wrote an e-mail to a good friend who faithfully prays for me and my health. I told her my situation, explained what I had done, and then wrote, "I promise I will control my eating the rest of the day and won't do something stupid like stop by Cinnabon and have a Mochalotta Chill when I'm at the mall." I suddenly felt more relaxed, had peace, and was in control of my eating the rest of the day.

Guidelines to Prevent "Stress Eating"

1. **Know why you are eating.** Proverbs 14:15 says, *"The simple believeth every word: but the prudent man looketh well to his going."* Are you truly hungry, or is it another stimuli causing you to eat?

4. **Recognize what other stimuli cause you to eat.** Are you a habit eater (where you "graze" all day long), stress eater, nervous eater, or a "see-food" eater (you see it so you eat it)?

3. **Make a plan.** Make a plan for what you will do when you realize you are eating in response to some stimuli other than truly being hungry—whether it is stress or just because the food is in front of you. Also make a plan to help prevent your feeling hungry. Had I taken a few minutes in the morning to plan my meals or had I packed some healthy snacks I could have prevented some of my frustration. Schedule and planning does a lot to help keep us on track.

STEP TWO PRINCIPLES

1. **Get seven to eight hours of uninterrupted sleep a night.**

2. **Learn to handle emotional stress in a Scriptural manner.** Walk with God. Praise Him. Exercise mind control. Thank God for everything in your life. Laugh a lot. Refuse to be easily offended. Take the necessary steps to prevent "stress eating."

Proper Exercise, Sunlight, and Oxygen

Moderate Exercise

Go to any garage sale, and you'll probably find a piece (or several pieces!) of "like-new" exercise equipment for sale! Most people realize that they should exercise, but the majority of people seldom do so.

Actually there are two extremes regarding exercise. The first group of people never exercises. The sum total of their daily exercise routine is picking up the remote control, walking to the refrigerator and back to the sofa during commercials! The second group of people over-exercise, many of whom are consumed with their exercise regimen.

Few people realize that it is possible to over-exercise. It is just as damaging to the metabolism to over-exert your body with exercise as it is to never exercise. Exercise is part of the "using up" cycle in our bodies. When we do extreme exercising, we tear down more than our bodies are able to rebuild. A common mind set regarding exercise is that "fast" and "more" is better. That is not so. Excessive exercise (whether in length or intensity) causes hormonal imbalances as your body uses up functional and structural biochemicals more than it is able to rebuild them. Over-exercising damages your metabolism.

The One Who created us left us a wonderful "owner's manual" to help us know how to take care of these bodies—*moderation, temperance,* and *temperate* are all words God used in the Bible as traits that should characterize our lives. In fact, *temperance* is listed in Galatians 5:22, 23, *"But the fruit of the Spirit is love, joy, peace, longsuffering, gentleness, goodness, faith, Meekness, temperance: against such there is no law."* One evidence of a Spirit-filled life is a life of temperance or moderation.

One can go to hundreds of medical Web sites on the Internet regarding exercise, and they all list the many benefits of moderate exercise. Moderate exercise helps to:

1. Reduce the risk of degenerative diseases such as arthritis, cancer, heart disease, hypertension, etc.
2. Increase energy levels
3. Improve sense of well-being
4. Improve quality of sleep
5. Improve bowel movements

6.   Lower cholesterol and blood-sugar levels
7.   Lower blood pressure
8.   Improve heart function
9.   Increase lean body tissue and reduce fat deposits, especially around the middle

As with almost anything, exercise can become an obsession. I know of ladies who exercise intensely for one to two hours a day seven days a week. Exercise should be done in moderation, not intensely. Mrs. Cindy Schaap suggests that ladies exercise for 20 to 30 minutes 4 to 5 times a week. She is a lady who keeps her body in balance and her priorities in order. I trust her advice implicitly. To keep my exercising a little more interesting, I walk some days and bicycle some days. When I choose to walk, I do not walk in a "near run"; I walk at a normal rate and walk about 2 miles in 30 minutes. Walking is a moderate exercise and is much healthier than jogging or a "run-walk" type of exercise. There is a "high" that a runner gets from exercising, but it takes its toll on the body as it causes the adrenal glands to secrete extra "feel good" hormones. This eventually depletes the body's supply and causes adrenal burnout. For more information on exercise, read Dr. Diana Swcharzbein's book, *The Schwarzbein Principle—The Program*. The exercise should be a tool to help heal our metabolism or to maintain a healthy metabolism. We should not

> The advantage of exercising every day is that you die healthier.

allow it to become an obsession or an addiction.

Exercise Tips

•   Though I never criticize anyone for doing so, I do not suggest that ladies go to fitness gyms, even if they are for women only. Oftentimes the atmosphere and the philosophies at these gyms are not pleasing to Christ.

•   Some of the best exercise costs little or nothing. Bicycling, roller blading, and walking are all relatively inexpensive and practical forms of exercise. If you have access to a swimming pool, swimming is also a great exercise.

•   Exercise at the same time every day. My friend and coworker, Linda Stubblefield, likes to ride her bike. (In the winter she uses indoor exercise equipment). I live on the same street as the Stubblefields and often see Linda and her husband David riding their bikes in the early evening. I, on the other hand, like to exercise early in the morning. I find that if I get up and exercise first thing in the morning, I am much more faithful at it than if I wait until later in the day. I have a niece who has two young boys. She walks every night after she has fixed dinner, cleaned up, and has things ready for the next day. Her husband leaves for work at 4:50 a.m. every day, so it is not practical for her to walk early in the morning. Just do what works best for you.

•   Keep safety in mind. In the winter when I walk early in the morning, it is still dark. Therefore, I have some inexpensive blinking lights I attach to my jacket so I can be easily spotted by drivers. When you walk, ride your bike, or roller blade, keep traffic in mind. Stay on the correct side of the road; try to listen for and be aware of traffic (coming from both directions).

• To prevent injuries, be sure you have the proper equipment and that the equipment is well maintained—comfortable walking shoes that give good support, bicycle tires with the proper amount of air, etc.

• Breathe deeply to keep the oxygen flowing to the cells.

• Do stretching exercises before and after you exercise.

• Drink plenty of water to keep your body hydrated. Dehydration requires your heart to pump harder for the blood to carry oxygen to the tissues.

• Eat a balanced diet so your body is getting the energy and nutrition it needs. Failing to eat enough food, skipping meals, etc. will negate the benefits of the exercise as you will be using up more biochemicals than you are replacing.

• Have a partner if you need one. My friend Carol Tudor has a young married lady who shows up every morning to go biking with her. She has said many times, "I know I won't do it if I'm not accountable to someone." Knowing that person is going to show up prevents her from talking herself out of biking each day.

• Have fun! Unless someone is walking with me, I use the time to pray, to praise God, or to work on Bible memory. I love taking in all the beauty of the season, whether it is all the beautiful flowers in the neatly manicured lawns on our street in the summer or the black silhouette of the trees against a brilliant sunrise in the middle of January.

> The most common exercise for women is jumping to conclusions.

Sunlight

Sunlight has received some bad publicity in recent years causing people to believe that it is very dangerous to get sunlight. The fact is, sunlight provides much-needed Vitamin D to your body and has many benefits. Consider the following report from the official BBC Internet Web site:

After years of adverse publicity, new research suggests that sunshine actually does bathe us in a favorable light after all. Scientists believe sunlight may reduce the risk of several types of cancer. Recent studies have found that sunlight can help protect you from cancer of the breast, colon, ovary, bladder, womb, stomach, and prostate gland.

The sun also provides us with our main source of vitamin D. Scientists have long been aware that this nutrient strengthens our bones and muscles and boosts the immune system. Ten minutes of daily exposure to sunlight will supply us with all the vitamin D that we need. The principal function of this vitamin is to promote calcium absorption in the gut and calcium transfer across cell membranes. This contributes to strong bones and a contented nervous system.

Low vitamin D is associated with several autoimmune diseases including multiple sclerosis, rheumatoid arthritis, thyroiditis, and Crohn's disease. Recent laboratory experiments suggest that vitamin D can also prevent the growth and spread of cancerous tumours.

Apart from the obvious positive associations we have with a sunny day, the sun can alter your mood chemically and even prevent depression. The onset of spring gives thousands of people relief from "seasonal affective disorder" or SAD. This miserable condition is a suppression of serotonin experienced by many who are deprived of sunlight during the dreary winter months.

Sunlight also stimulates the pineal gland, a tiny pea-sized organ found in the base of the brain. Sometimes known as "the third eye," the pineal gland produces certain types of chemicals called tryptamines. One type of tryptamine, melatonin, keeps our body clock aware of night and day and the changing seasons.[1]

> My mother started walking 5 miles a day when she was 60. She's 97 now, and we have no idea where she is.

Just 10 minutes of exposure to sunlight a day brings many benefits to the body. What most people don't realize is that diseases such as cancer are a result of a damaged metabolism and a weakened immune system. The diseases are caused from within not from without. Brushing and flossing one's teeth are important, but neither are the best preventive for tooth decay. Healthy teeth are best maintained by good nutrition. (Since changing my eating habits nearly ten years ago and adding Barley Max to my daily regimen, I have not had one new cavity. I have had some fillings come out that needed to be replaced but no new cavities.) The best preventive for skin cancer is not staying out of the sun; it is a nutritious, balanced diet. Cancer is an immune system problem.

Oxygen

The most vital nutrient our body requires is oxygen. While a person can go for several days without water and several weeks without food, one can only go a few minutes without oxygen before brain damage or death occurs.

Every living person is a breathing person and gets oxygen into the body, but few people breathe deeply and exercise in a way that provides the oxygen our bodies need to be healthy. Breathing has two parts: inhaling (breathing in) and exhaling (breathing out). Inhaling is the only means we have to provide our bodies and its various organs with the supply of oxygen which is vital for our survival. Exhaling is one means to get rid of waste products and toxins from the body.

The brain requires more oxygen than any other organ. When the brain does not get enough oxygen, the result is mental sluggishness, negative thoughts and depression, and eventually vision and hearing decline. That is why older people and those whose arteries are clogged often become senile because oxygen to the brain is reduced. Poor oxygen supply affects all parts of the body. Probably you will recall the mining accident in West Virginia in the spring of 2006. All of the men trapped in the mine died except for one. The man who lived suffers from a number of problems because his body was deprived of the oxygen it needed for an extended period of time.

For a long time, lack of oxygen has been considered a major cause of cancer. As far back as 1947, work done in Germany showed that when oxygen was withdrawn, normal body cells could turn into cancer cells. Cancer cannot survive in an oxygen rich environment. Studies also show that rich supplies of oxygen help prevent heart attacks, strokes, and other diseases. Thus, oxygen is very critical to our well-being, and any effort to increase the supply of oxygen to our body and especially to the brain will pay rich dividends.

Breathing exercises are particularly important for people who have sedentary jobs and spend most of the day in offices. Their brains are oxygen starved, and their bodies are just "getting by." Do you ever wonder why you feel tired, nervous, and irritable or seem to be counterproductive after you have been sitting at a desk working for an extended period of time? A lack of oxygen to the cells is one of the main causes of these symptoms. In addition to that, the immune system is affected, making a person more susceptible colds, flu, and other "bugs."

One of the major keys to vitality and rejuvenation is a purified blood stream. Since oxygen purifies the blood stream, the quickest and most effective way to purify the blood stream is by taking in extra supplies of oxygen from the air we breathe. Good breathing exercises are the most effective method for saturating the blood with extra oxygen. By purifying the blood stream, every part of the body benefits, including the mind. Your complexion will become clearer and brighter, and wrinkles will begin to fade away.

Simple breathing exercises can be done almost anywhere, and you will reap great benefits to your body while you increase your energy levels and experience renewed vitality. Oftentimes when you feel sleepy during the day, your body is signaling that you need more oxygen (though sometimes it can be a signal that your blood sugar is low, and you need food).

For most of us, our inhaling is too shallow, which prevents our lungs (and hence, our cells) from getting the oxygen they need to function properly. Then our exhal-

> A gym teacher instructed a lady to touch her toes. She said, "I don't have that kind of relationship with my feet. Can I just wave?"

ing is also too shallow, which fails to get rid of the toxins, leaving carbon dioxide in our lungs. Our lungs need exercise; breathing deeply and slowly will meet that need.

The benefits of breathing deeply and getting the necessary oxygen to the cells are numerous. They include:

- Assists with weight loss (extra oxygen helps burn fat more efficiently)
- Improves blood quality which aids in the elimination of toxins from our systems
- Aids in the digestion of food and causes the digestive system to work more efficiently.
- Improves the health of the nervous system, including the brain, spinal cord, nerve centers and nerves which helps the entire body since the nervous system communicates to all parts of the body.
- Rejuvenates the glands, especially the pituitary and pineal glands (located in the brain). The brain requires three times more oxygen than does the rest of the body.
- Helps the skin become smoother and reduces facial wrinkles.
- Contributes to healthy lungs which helps prevent respiratory problems.
- Reduces the work load for the heart which results in a more efficient, stronger heart.
- Helps reduce blood pressure.
- Relaxes the mind and the body.

Below is an exercise that will help you to deepen your breathing, cleanse your lungs, increase your energy, and decrease tension. Practice this exercise about five minutes several times a day—especially when you are feeling sleepy or irritable, or are experiencing a lack of concentration.

1. Sit up straight. Exhale.
2. Inhale through your nose. At the same time, relax the abdominal muscles. It should feel as though the abdomen is filling with air.
3. After filling the belly, keep inhaling and fill up the middle of your chest. You will feel your chest and rib cage expand.
4. Hold the breath in while you slowly count to five, and then begin to exhale as slowly as possible.
5. As the air is slowly let out through your mouth, relax your chest and rib cage. Begin to pull your belly in to force out the remaining breath.
6. Close your eyes, let everything go, and concentrate solely on your breathing.

> They keep telling us to get in touch with our bodies. Mine isn't all that chatty, but the other day I asked it, "Body, how'd you like to go to the 6:00 a.m. class in vigorous toning?" Clear as a bell my body said, "Listen, girl-friend…do it, and you die."

7.   Relax your face and mind.

Another principle to keep in mind regarding getting proper amounts of oxygen to your cells is proper posture. When we sit in a "slouched" position or lie in bed at night in that type of position, we do not breathe properly and, therefore, deprive our lungs of much-needed oxygen. Whether sitting or standing, keep your shoulders up and back to help your breathing process.

STEP THREE PRINCIPLES

- Schedule a moderate exercise program for 20 to 30 minutes four to five times a week.
- Try to get 10 minutes of sunlight every day.
- Practice deep breathing exercises for three to five minutes several times a day.

Setting Goals

During the last session of a teaching workshop, participants were asked to state their personal goals for the immediate future. One teacher vowed to update photo albums, another to lose weight. The goal that got the most response, however, was given by a slightly out-of-shape kindergarten teacher. "I resolve to exercise until I can complete a 20-minute workout in less than an hour," she said.

Proper Elimination of Toxic Chemicals

Toxic Chemicals: A Detriment to a Healthy Metabolism

Toxic chemicals have a very negative effect on our metabolism and accelerate the aging process in our bodies. Most toxic chemicals give temporary boosts of energy that fool the body into thinking it has more energy and that the body is healthier than it actually is. These toxic chemicals actually "rewire" your body chemistry for a short-term boost, but in the end, they leave your system disoriented and out of balance. They do not help the body rebuild; rather, they use up, which, of course, damages your metabolism.

Though all of the following are toxic chemicals and therefore are damaging to your metabolism, there are degrees of damage that they do. (But keep in mind *all* of them are toxic to your body, and all damage your metabolism!) I have listed them in order of the degree of damage they do. Therefore, the higher on the list the chemical is positioned, the more damaging that particular chemical is to your metabolism.

1. **Illicit drugs and narcotics.** Our bodies have their own natural "feel-good" chemicals that are released into the blood stream. For example, when a person exercises, the brain releases chemicals called endorphins which are actually mood enhancers; they lift a person's spirit. Illicit drugs and narcotics cause our body to release its own natural mood enhancing chemicals in much higher quantities than normal. However, when the chemicals are gone, the person is left listless and depressed—leaving the body craving more. Illicit drugs are extremely addicting.

2. **Tobacco/Nicotine.** Nicotine is a stimulant that takes its toll on your body by decreasing appetite and by increasing blood pressure and heart rate. The diseases caused by tobacco are staggering: cancer, heart attacks, strokes, emphysema, depression, allergies, acid reflux, osteoporosis, and dementia to name a few.

3. **Alcohol.** In addition to the fact that liquor limits a person's ability to think clearly and also affects the use of one's motor skills (wreaking havoc in homes, in people's personal lives, and on the road with numbers of terrible injuries and deaths each year), it poses several problems to the metabolism. The first problem with alcohol is that

is causes cell death. It destroys cells in the brain (and I really don't know anyone who can afford to lose brain cells!). The second problem alcohol causes to the metabolism is that the sugar content of alcohol increases the release of insulin. Alcohol use causes diseases such as diabetes, obesity, cirrhosis of the liver, heart disease, high blood pressure, and coronary artery disease.

4. **Prescription and over-the-counter drugs.** The body uses orthomolecules to carry out many of its functions. Ingesting medications causes orthomolecules to be displaced by foreign substances. Though drugs often help one part of the body, most medications cause side effects that are just as bad or worse than the problem being treated. Dr. Dennis Streeter, a Christian physician who attends our church, says, "Drugs mask the problem by treating the symptoms." Therefore, we are better off not using any drugs at all if we can help it. *Warning: Do not stop taking any prescription drugs without first consulting your primary care physician.* Though most drugs are harmful to the metabolism, you cannot stop using them cold turkey, especially if you have not fixed the underlying problem for which they were prescribed in the first place.

Drugs are meant to help a myriad of symptoms, but the side effects of drugs (even over-the-counter drugs) are very damaging to the body. They include liver damage, brain damage, colon problems, cancer, insomnia, depression, personality changes, mood swings, heart attacks, and more. It is important that you read the side effects of any drug before taking it, whether it is a prescription drug or an over-the-counter medication. There are many natural supplements that you can take as alternatives to over-the-counter drugs.

Warning: Please be aware of the drug interaction that can be caused by taking supplements. Do your research!

Allow me to give you a personal illustration as to the importance of knowing how supplements can affect medications you are taking. A friend told me she had been taking calcium and a daily multiple vitamin for about a year and how much better she felt. I thought, "I can do that," and so I began taking a calcium tablet and a good multi-vitamin every day. After taking the calcium for about four months, I realized that many of my old hypothyroid symptoms were reappearing—dry hair, fatigue, weight gain, etc. A few days later I finished my bottles of calcium and the multi-vitamin and went to the cupboard to get new ones. I

Ice Cream Flavors

The young man entered the Ice Cream Palace and asked, "What kinds of ice cream do you have?"

"Vanilla, chocolate, strawberry," the girl wheezed as she spoke, patted her chest, and seemed unable to continue.

"Do you have laryngitis?" the young man asked sympathetically.

"Nope," she whispered, "just vanilla, chocolate, and strawberry."

thought to myself, "I seem to feel worse since I started taking these instead of better." But I shook it off and decided to keep on taking them. When I got a haircut a few weeks later, my hair stylist said, "Are you still taking your thyroid medication?" I told her I was, and she said, "Your hair is looking like it did before you started on thyroid medication. I agreed with her, but I wasn't sure what to do about it.

While working on this book, I visited Barnes & Noble to look at books on women's health (something I do regularly) and saw a book entitled, *Living Well With Hypothyroidism.* I decided to peruse the book and happened to noticed a headline about calcium. I was shocked to read that taking thyroid medication with calcium reduces the absorption rate of the thyroid medication by nearly 50 percent! In other words, I had only been absorbing a little more than half of my thyroid medication! The author said it is imperative to take your calcium at least four hours *after* ingesting thyroid medication so the calcium does not block the absorption of the medicine. I immediately made the advised change the next day, and though I can tell a difference, it will probably take several months to repair the damage that was done. Taking calcium *with* my thyroid medication for nearly six months caused my body to be robbed of much-needed thyroid medication for that period of time.

If you do take supplements, be well read and know how they may interact with drugs you may be taking and also how they interact with each other. Be responsible even with natural supplements!

5. Artificial sweeteners. The average American believes artificial sweeteners are a healthy choice, but they are actually toxic to the body. They are chemicals, so they are not recognized as useable food for the body. They also stimulate the appetite, causing a person to want to eat more. Artificial sweeteners include aspartame, sucralose, saccharine, acesulfam-K. Artificial sweeteners do not make diet

> One of life's mysteries is how a two-pound box of candy can make a woman gain five pounds.

> Because of an ear infection, little Johnny had to go to the pediatrician. The doctor directed his comments and questions to little Johnny in a professional manner. When he asked, "Is there anything you are allergic to?" little Johnny nodded and whispered in his ear.
>
> Smiling, the pediatrician wrote out a prescription and handed it to little Johnny's mother. She tucked it into her purse without looking at it. As the pharmacist filled the order, he remarked on the unusual food-drug interaction little Johnny must have.
>
> Little Johnny's mother looked puzzled until he showed her the label on the bottle. As per the doctor's instructions, it read, "Do not take with broccoli."

beverages (even decaffeinated sodas) a wise choice.

6. Refined sugars. Of course, sugar in any form stimulates the pancreas. A diet that includes a lot of refined sugars leads to diabetes, heart disease, strokes, etc. Refined sugars include white sugar, brown sugar, sucrose, fructose, maltose, dextrose, maltodextrin, polydextrose, corn syrup, and high fructose corn syrup. There are many foods that contain hidden sugars such as milk (especially skim milk) and fruit juice. Read the labels on foods before you buy them. You'll be quite surprised at the amount of sugar in foods, including salad dressing, condiments, junk food, bread, etc.

7. Additives, chemical preservatives, and other chemicals. It has been said that when reading the ingredients on the label of foods you are about to purchase, "If you can't pronounce it, you probably shouldn't be eating it!" MSG (monosodium glutamate) is one of the more well-known additives in food that causes problems for people, but all of the man-made chemicals that are added to food for flavor and preservation interfere with hormone messaging. This includes fake fats such as Olestra. These products are man-made. Your body cannot use these chemicals to repair or rebuild. One good thing about these additives and preservatives is that while most toxic chemicals are very addicting, these are not, so

> Drink coffee. Do stupid things faster and with more energy.

you will not experience any type of withdrawal symptoms.

8. Caffeine. Found in beverages such as coffee, soda, and some teas (black and green), caffeine stimulates the adrenal glands, so it supplies some temporary high energy. Caffeine is addicting, and it also causes the body to use up its chemicals faster than it rebuilds them. If you enjoy the taste of coffee, you can do so without the damaging effects of caffeine by drinking organic Swiss water processed decaf coffee. This should be used in moderation, but the Swiss water process removes most of the caffeine without the use of harsh chemicals. Most decaffeinated coffee goes through a chemical process that makes the decaffeinated coffee just as damaging to the metabolism as regular coffee because of the chemicals. It is best to "wean" off of coffee rather than try to quit "cold turkey."

Please note the following facts regarding toxic chemicals:

1. Generally, people use toxic chemicals to feel better or to get more accomplished when they feel stressed or are not eating properly. These substances help with mood, concentration, and give a feeling of well-being.

2. For that reason, outside of additives and chemical preservatives, *toxic chemicals are addicting;* they are an artificial way to make you feel better temporarily. The fact that these toxic chemicals are addicting makes anyone using them

a prime target for the Devil to build a stronghold in their life. (Strongholds are addictions.)

3. Because toxic chemicals are addictive, it is very difficult to stop using these chemicals "cold turkey" without changing the reasons you started using them in the first place. That is why proper food choices and proper sleep are a must before trying to remove the toxic chemicals from your lifestyle.

4. Oftentimes people believe that using sugar substitutes instead of sugar is being good to their bodies. Both are toxic chemicals, so a sugar substitute really is not part of a healthy lifestyle.

5. Often people take drugs that are supposed to help their health (such as insulin or cholesterol-lowering drugs) and fail to work on the root problem that caused the diseases in the first place.

The most important change that will better enable you to get off of toxic chemicals is good nutrition. Eating three balanced meals and one or two snacks (consisting of protein, healthy fat, non-starchy vegetables, and real carbohydrates such as fruit and whole grains) throughout the day will help ease the uncontrollable craving for chemicals such as sugar and caffeine.

Another way to help ease the cravings and to wean off the toxic chemicals is to replace more dangerous chemicals with less toxic ones. For example, if you are very addicted to refined sugar, try the following:

- Eat berries and grapefruit with whole-fat whipping cream.
- Eat small amounts of bitter, dark chocolate.
- Substitute caffeinated coffee, black tea, or green tea for refined sugars.
- Of course, your goal is to get off of all toxic chemicals but use less harmful chemicals to help you in the transition while you improve your nutrition.

A second key to help you get off of toxic chemicals is to get proper sleep. One of the reasons people ingest toxic chemicals such as sugar and caffeine in the first place is to have more energy. However, the best way to have more energy is to rebuild energy during sleep, not break down healthy tissues by using toxic chemicals.

Getting off of toxic chemicals is not the first step in healing your metabolism. Eating properly, sleeping well, and managing stress come first. But the goal is to get off of the toxic chemicals as soon as you are able to do so. It probably will not be an easy task, but the more diligent you are in eating the proper foods and in getting the proper rest, the easier it will be for you.

It is easy to observe that drinking alcohol, partaking in recreational drugs, or smoking cigarettes is sin. They are considered a part of the world's system and preached against as an issue of separation from the world. However, substances such as sugar are very addictive and do great damage to the body. They accelerate

Three little words that mean so much—
SOLID MILK CHOCOLATE

the aging process and damage our metabolism. The greatest reason we have to be concerned about the aging process is that the healthier we are, the more we are able to do for God. How can we do less than take care of the body He has given us so we can, in great gratitude, serve Him with all our strength?

Romans 12:1 says, *"I beseech you therefore, brethren, by the mercies of God, that ye present your bodies a living sacrifice, holy, acceptable unto God, which is your reasonable service."* That would include weaning off of toxic chemicals.

If you are addicted to toxic chemicals and it has become a stronghold in your life, you will want to read the last unit in this book and follow the advice given on those pages (including the recommended reading).

Estrogen Dominance and Toxic Chemicals

Estrogen dominance deals with hormones which will be discussed in the next chapter, but it is so related to the problem of toxic chemicals that I decided to include it with this chapter. One of the more common causes of hormone imbalance today is estrogen dominance, a term coined by the late Dr. John Lee who was a pioneer in women's health and bioidentical hormone replacement. There are a number of different hormone issues that can

> Inside of me there's a thin person struggling to get out, but I can usually sedate her with four or five cupcakes.

occur in the human body, but I want to address the reproductive hormones in this section—and more specifically estrogen dominance.

There are substances in our environment called xenohormones (also sometimes called xenoestrogens). These are synthetic chemicals such as pesticides and plastics which have toxic influences on all living creatures. Xenohormones have the same molecular makeup as estrogen. Therefore, when our bodies ingest xenohormones—whether through foods we eat, the air we breath, or through our skin—our estrogen receptors cannot tell the difference between the estrogen our bodies produce and the xenohormones.

Xenohormones are everywhere! They are in dish and laundry detergents, makeup, hairstyling products, pesticides, insecticides, in plastic (including all the plastic food containers in which we purchase and store food), and in cleaning supplies to name a few. These xenohormones have an impact on the state of our health and especially influence our hormones.

All of these xenohormones coming into our bodies causes *estrogen dominance*. Some of the causes of estrogen dominance include poor diet, stress, birth control pills, conventional hormone replacement therapy, and environmental issues.

Following are some of the symptoms and diseases caused by estrogen dominance:
- Breast cancer
- Breast tenderness

- Cervical dysplasia
- Cold hands and feet
- Copper excess
- Decreased sex drive
- Depression with anxiety or agitation
- Dry eyes
- Early onset of menstruation
- Endometrial (uterine) cancer
- Fat gain, especially around the abdomen, hips and thighs
- Fatigue
- Fibrocystic breasts
- Fibromyalgia
- Foggy thinking
- Gallbladder disease
- Hair loss
- Headaches
- Hypoglycemia
- Increased blood clotting (increasing stroke risk)
- Infertility
- Insulin resistance
- Irregular menstrual periods
- Irritability
- Insomnia
- Joint pain
- Magnesium deficiency
- Memory loss
- Mood swings
- Muscle pain
- Obesity
- Osteoporosis
- PMS
- Polycystic ovaries
- Premenopausal bone loss
- Sluggish metabolism
- Suicidal feelings
- Thyroid dysfunction mimicking hypothyroidism
- Uterine cancer
- Uterine fibroids
- Water retention, bloating
- Zinc deficiency[1]

These symptoms are not limited to women going through menopause. Estrogen dominance is affecting the health of women of all ages (and I might add the health of men also.)

Women's Reproductive Hormones

God created a woman's body to be able to reproduce and bring babies into the world. To make that happen, He gave us reproductive hormones, specifically estrogen (actually three estrogens including estrone, estrodial, and estriol), progesterone, and testosterone being the main ones. (Men have the exact same hormones women have, but they have different proportions.) God designed a very complex and beautiful system.

Estrogen creates cellular proliferation; it makes cells grow very, very quickly. Estrogen is what turns a little girl into a woman. When

> They call it PMS because Mad Cow Disease was already taken.

God made woman, He knew that the estrogen the body produces requires balance; the body cannot have cells grow and grow without something to balance them out. Progesterone is the hormone that is the "balancing act" for estrogen. If your body was a car, we could compare estrogen to the gas pedal and progesterone to the brakes. A car that goes without having brakes gets into big trouble. Many women today are estrogen dominant with not enough progesterone to balance out all that estrogen. In other words, there is lots of "gas" with no "brakes."

Allow me to explain the monthly cycle of a premenopausal woman. During the first half of a 28-day cycle, the body produces primarily the estrogens, and during the last half of the cycle, the body produces primarily progesterone. During the first half of the cycle, the estrogen (causing cellular proliferation) builds a soft, thick lining on the wall of the uterus in preparation for pregnancy. The uterus is about the size of a large orange or a small grapefruit. Meanwhile, the ovarian follicles begin developing an egg. Near the middle of the cycle, estrogen production peaks and begins to taper off as the follicle matures and the egg is released from the ovaries. The egg travels down the fallopian tubes, and if it is fertilized, it attaches to the wall of the uterus in that nice, soft, thick lining. When the egg is released (called ovulation), the follicle becomes what is called the *corpus luteum,* which is the site of progesterone production. Progesterone is the hormone that dominates in the last half of the cycle. One function of the progesterone is to keep that egg on the wall. It is an anti-spasmodic and prevents the uterus from going into spasms. If the uterus goes into spasms, the baby automatically aborts. (There is a small section on infertility at the end of the next chapter.)

If the egg is not fertilized, the progesterone takes on a completely different role. Its job at that point is to get rid of and clean out all of those layers in your uterus. Therefore, progesterone production slows drastically. Since progesterone is an anti-spasmodic, when the production slows, the uterus goes into spasms and menstruation begins.

Estrogen and progesterone need to be balanced in a proper ratio. They should be doing a nice little "dance" every month as I explained in the previous paragraphs. However, all of the petrochemicals, plastics, etc. which have estrogen-like qualities, make our estrogen levels high. The higher the estrogen levels get, the more out-of-balance our bodies become, and the more we find women plagued with PMS, endometriosis, infertility, and so forth. How did this estrogen dominance happen?

1. **Petroleum-based products—petrochemicals.** Before World War II the United States was not a petroleum-based country. But plastic—a petroleum-based product—was developed, and we have since become a petroleum-based society.

> I used to think chocolate was bad for you, so I stopped thinking.

Petroleum-based products have a molecular structure that fits like a lock and key into our receptors.

A woman's body has two ovaries about the size of a walnut on either side of the uterus. The primary function of the ovum is to produce eggs and hormones. When the body is in balance and the hormones function as they are supposed to, the ovaries produce progesterone, and the progesterone, estrogens, and testosterone attach to the receptors. When these hormones attach the way they are supposed to, the body is in perfect hormone balance. When these hormones are in balance, you don't experience PMS, fibrocystic breasts, fibroid tumors, and all of the other difficult symptoms associated with reproductive hormone imbalances.

However, when the body ingests xenohormones, they attach to the receptors. They are not really estrogens, but they function like estrogens because of their molecular structure. The receptors don't know the difference between the body's estrogens and the xenoestrogens because the molecular structure is identical. Because xenohormones fit onto the receptors, when progesterone tries to attach to the receptor it is unable to do so because the receptors are filled with xenoestrogens. The progesterone has no place to go, so the body binds it with a protein and carries it out through the blood stream. When this happens day after day, the progesterone levels get lower and lower. That is one reason why there are so many female hormone issues in our country.

Because of the excessive amounts of estrogen and the lack of progesterone, their hormones are terribly out of balance and those women suffer from many of the symptoms listed above.

2. Growth Hormones in Animals.
Another cause of estrogen dominance is the hormones administered to animals. This was a practice started in the 1960s. Why are growth hormones given to animals? Money! Estrogen makes cellular proliferation which causes the animals to grow quickly and gets them to market sooner. It's all about money. Dairy cattle are also given hormones (a form of estrogen) to cause them to produce greater amounts of milk.

The public is told by government officials that these hormones are safe, but if that is true, why is it that the average age for a girl to start her period was 14.3 and today it is 10.7 (and 9.2 among African Americans). Children are entering puberty at 9 and 10 years of age! Numbers of boys look like they are developing breasts. The number of overweight children is at an all-time high. It surely seems that all of the hormones in meat and dairy products must play some role in this change.

3. Surgically Induced Menopause. There are times when a hysterectomy is needed for health reasons—cancer or a prolapsed uterus are the two main reasons. When a woman experiences problems with her reproductive organs, unless she has can-

> If you drink a diet soda with a candy bar, the calories in the candy bar are canceled out by the diet soda.

cer or a prolapsed uterus, she should take the following thoughts into consideration before agreeing to have a hysterectomy. It is commonly thought that once a woman's reproductive years are ended, she has no need for a uterus, but that is not the case.

Evidence shows that the uterus plays a role in immune function—it produces the prostaglandins responsible for a variety of physiological functions. The uterus helps in prevention of cardiovascular disease through the production of prostacyclin, which prevents blood clots. The uterus also secretes a small amount of estrogen. Women who have had hysterectomies also appear to be at increased risk of osteoporosis and osteoarthritis. [A] hysterectomy also impacts libido: for some women, the removal of the uterus causes an abrupt end to her sex drive. In fact, particularly in the case of [a] hysterectomy due to [a] prolapsed uterus, research shows that 50 percent of hysterectomies end sexual intercourse permanently. The reason for this can be due to the surgeon damaging nerves or inhibiting blood flow to the clitoris or pelvic region.[2]

Is it any wonder that heart disease, low libido, and other health issues are such common problems with women who've had hysterectomies? **Never agree to a hysterectomy (getting rid of your uterus) without taking the health benefits of your uterus into consideration.** How much better to make necessary lifestyle changes first to try and remedy your symptoms than to rush into surgery and later experience a whole set of other symptoms as a result. I had a hysterectomy long before I heard of prostacyclin and its benefits to the body. Considering that both of my parents and all four of my grandparents suffered from heart disease, I wish I'd had the benefit of knowing about this important chemical before I agreed to my hysterectomy.

There is another issue to consider when deciding to have a hysterectomy with the removal of the ovaries (the ovaries are not always removed with a hysterectomy), as it relates to xenoestrogens in the body. Once the ovaries are removed, the body no longer produces progesterone.

Progesterone is a precursor (building block) for most other hormones including DHEA, estradiol, testosterone and cortisol. Progesterone, like estradiol, plays an important role in mood, blood-sugar balance, sex drive, and thyroid function, as well as adrenal gland health.[3]

Therefore, removal of the ovaries greatly affects the production of other hormones since progesterone is the building block for those hormones.

> Customer to Waiter:
> "I'm going to order a salad and the broiled, skinless chicken breast, but I want you to bring me lasagna and garlic bread by mistake."

Also, since progesterone is the "balancing act" for estrogen and because progesterone is produced by the ovaries, the body has no way to produce the adequate amount of progesterone the body needs if the ovaries are removed.

4. Traditional Hormone Replacement Therapy and Chemical Birth Control. As ladies in their forties (sometimes earlier) begin to experience symptoms of menopause, it is common for their physicians to prescribe what is referred to as hormone replacement therapy (HRT). There has been much controversy as to the real benefit as well as the negative side effects of HRT. The biggest problem with traditional HRT is that the estrogen replacement is actually a xenoestrogen rather than a bioidentical estrogen. (This difference will be more fully explained in the next chapter.) Therefore, traditional HRT actually contributes to estrogen dominance rather than helping to balance your hormones.

5. Poor Nutrition. The importance of a balanced diet of real foods has been indicated clearly previously in this book. Therefore, I will not present a lengthy argument in this paragraph. Eating processed foods which are filled with chemicals and refined sugar contributes greatly to estrogen dominance.

Reducing Estrogen Dominance

Estrogen dominance is a real problem that is affecting the entire population of our nation. We owe it to the next generation to make changes to protect them and to help them repair some of the damage that has been done. These changes have to start with you and me. What can we do?

All of these xenoestrogens are actually toxic chemicals and should be treated as such following the guidelines listed in the earlier part of this chapter. Some additional thoughts:

• It is important at this point to emphasize again that food choices are very important in helping to get rid of toxic chemicals since so many foods contain chemicals and hormones. Keep in mind that a number of animal products including cattle dairy products contain growth hormones. (Goat and buffalo dairy products are much more environmental and body friendly, as is buffalo meat. I thought it sounded a little too "out of the loop" for me, but some friends took me to an upscale restaurant that served buffalo steak. It was delicious, and I have since had buffalo burgers and buffalo chili, all of which are very good. Actually, it tastes to me like a really good cut of beef.)

Weight Watching

Having lost weight over the past few years, a lady was discarding things from her wardrobe that no longer fit. Her seven-year-old niece was watching as she held up a huge skirt. "Wow," the lady said, "I must have worn this when I was 253."

Her niece looked puzzled, then asked, "How old are you now?"

• Begin to replace the xenohormones (chemicals) you use in your home. Don't try to do it all at once as it can soon prove to be over-whelming. Make small changes as you are able to do so. Some changes you could do gradually are: change over to detergents that have no chemicals (these are available through some multi-level marketing companies and also at health food stores; be discretionary, as some of these just do not do the job while others are more effective than their chemical counterparts), discontinue the use of dryer sheets, eliminate dry cleaning as much as possible (any clothes which are dry cleaned should be aired out for 24 to 48 hours before putting them in the closet—airing outside is best), and so forth. Just making one change a month would mean 12 changes in a year, and each of those changes will help eliminate some of the toxic chemicals from your lifestyle.

• Bioidentical progesterone supplementation is a change that has literally helped thousands of women. Bioidentical progesterone is a cream that should be applied to the tender areas of your skin such as the abdomen, inner thighs,

Sugar Worry

A nurse at a hospital received a call from an anxious patient. "I'm a diabetic, and I'm afraid I've had too much sugar today," the caller said.

"Are you light-headed?" the nurse asked.

"No," the caller answered, "I'm a brunette."

breasts, etc. It is important that the bioidentical progesterone you use is free of petrochemicals. You can get "natural" or bioidentical progesterone at most health food stores. There are usually a number of brands to choose from. In the book, *What Your Doctor May Not Tell You About Menopause* there is a list of brands that are wise choices in bioidentical progesterone from health food stores. The brand of progesterone I use is listed in the "Resources" Appendix. One advantage of the brand I use is that it comes in a "pump" container. (The brands I previously used came with a small "scoop" for dispensing, but I have found the pump so much easier and practical.) Taking bioidentical progesterone can be one of the easiest fixes available for balancing out your estrogen/progesterone ratio. It has helped ladies with depression, low libido, and a number of other symptoms. Keep in mind that it is not a "magic potion" to cure all of your problems. Adding progesterone without changing poor eating habits or other lifestyle issues will not solve your health problems. However, I have had several women say to me, "My husband wants to be sure I keep an extra container of progesterone on hand at all times so I never run out!"

I have also had men simply say to me, "Thanks for helping my wife," after their wives started taking bioidentical progesterone. It is important to use bioidentical hormone replacement so the molecular structure is the same as the body's own ovaries make. That is why there are no side effects and why it is so successful. You will want to read the next chapter entitled, "Proper Hormone Replacement If Needed" before starting on natural progesterone. Avoid the philosophy, "If a little is good, a lot is better." A surplus of progesterone in your body is a hormonal imbalance just as a shortages.

STEP FOUR PRINCIPLES

1. Define the toxic chemicals that are a part of your lifestyle.

2. Take the necessary steps to begin eliminating the toxic chemicals, beginning with the most toxic.

3. Be sure to institute the first three steps in this unit. Taking care of these first three steps will enable you to more efficiently rid your lifestyle of the toxic chemicals.

- Proper nutrition and elimination
- Proper sleep and stress management
- Proper exercise, sunlight, and oxygen

4. If you are estrogen dominant, begin applying bioidentical progesterone cream.

Fast-Food Employee to Customer:

"If you'd like a healthy alternative, we can wrap your cheeseburger, French fries, and fruit pie in a low-fat tortilla."

Proper Hormone Replacement

The final phase, if needed, toward healing the metabolism is bioidentical hormone replacement. Some women, especially those whose symptoms are mild find that making changes in their food choices is all that is needed to get them back on track. Other women find they need to do several other steps outlined in this unit. There are numbers of women, however, who have hormone imbalances that the first four steps will not fix and who find they need to be on some type of hormone replacement. If you already know you have a hormone imbalance or suspect that you do, it is wise to be tested to begin your hormone replacement therapy as soon as possible.

Dr. Peter Ellis, a researcher at Harvard University, states that up to 85 percent of women in the United States have a hormone imbalance. If, after instituting the first four principles for healing your metabolism and if one or more of your hormonal systems is not functioning properly, you are among that 85 percent. When your body can no longer produce a certain hormone, it must be replaced so your metabolism can become balanced.

There are a myriad of symptoms for hormone imbalances, and the symptoms help indicate which hormones are lacking or missing. Following is a hormone balance "test" to help you learn if you should be tested for a hormone imbalance. This questionnaire is from the ZRT Laboratory Web site which uses both saliva and blood spot testing for hormones. (Some hormones are more accurately tested with a saliva sample than blood.)I have had my hormone testing done at ZRT Laboratory because that is the lab my physician uses. Several companies are listed in Appendix B on page 150, or you can go on the Internet to find a lab for testing. Do your research, however, to be sure the company you choose is a reputable company.

Keep in mind that this "test" is not for medical diagnosis purposes. Rather, it is a simple test to give you an idea if there is a possibility that you are experiencing a hormone imbalance. Once you decide to have the testing done, (you will need to go online to get a testing kit) you will need to take the test results to a physician for an accurate reading and for proper hormone replacement if necessary.

Directions:

1. Read carefully through the list of symptoms in each group and put a check mark next to each symptom that you have. (If you check the same symptom in more than one group, that's fine.)

2. Go back and count the check marks in each group. In any group where you have two or more symptoms checked, there's a good chance that you have the hormone imbalance represented by that group.

3. The more symptoms you check, the higher the likelihood that you have the hormone imbalance represented by that group. (Some people may have more than one type of hormonal imbalance.)

Hormone Balance Test for Women

SYMPTOM GROUP 1

- ❏ PMS
- ❏ Insomnia
- ❏ Early miscarriage
- ❏ Painful and/or lumpy breasts
- ❏ Unexplained weight gain
- ❏ Cyclical headaches
- ❏ Anxiety
- ❏ Infertility

_____ TOTAL BOXES CHECKED

(If you have checked two or more boxes in this group, turn to page 113 to learn what type of hormonal imbalance you may have.)

SYMPTOM GROUP 2

- ❏ Vaginal dryness
- ❏ Night sweats
- ❏ Painful intercourse
- ❏ Memory problems
- ❏ Bladder infections
- ❏ Lethargic depression
- ❏ Hot flashes

_____ TOTAL BOXES CHECKED

(If you have checked two or more boxes in this group, turn to page 114 to learn what type of hormonal imbalance you may have.)

SYMPTOM GROUP 3

- ❏ Puffiness and bloating
- ❏ Cervical dysplasia (abnormal pap smear)
- ❏ Rapid weight gain
- ❏ Breast tenderness
- ❏ Mood swings
- ❏ Heavy bleeding
- ❏ Anxious depression
- ❏ Migraine headaches
- ❏ Insomnia
- ❏ Foggy thinking
- ❏ Red flush on face
- ❏ Gallbladder problems
- ❏ Weepiness

_____ TOTAL BOXES CHECKED

(If you have checked two or more boxes in this group, turn to page 114 to learn what type of hormonal imbalance you may have.)

SYMPTOM GROUP 4

A combination of the symptoms in Symptom Group #1 and Symptom Group #3

_____ TOTAL BOXES CHECKED

(If you have checked two or more boxes in this group, turn to page 114 to learn what type of hormonal imbalance you may have.)

SYMPTOM GROUP 5

☐ Acne
☐ Polycystic ovary syndrome (PCOS)
☐ Excessive hair on the face and arms
☐ Hypoglycemia and/or unstable blood sugar
☐ Thinning hair on the head
☐ Infertility
☐ Ovarian cysts
☐ Mid-cycle pain

_____ TOTAL BOXES CHECKED

(If you have checked two or more boxes in this group, turn to page 114 to learn what type of hormonal imbalance you may have.)

SYMPTOM GROUP 6

☐ Debilitating fatigue
☐ Unstable blood sugar
☐ Foggy thinking
☐ Low blood pressure
☐ Thin and/or dry skin
☐ Intolerance to exercise
☐ Brown spots on face

_____ TOTAL BOXES CHECKED

(If you have checked two or more boxes in this group, turn to page 114 to learn what type of hormonal imbalance you may have.)

Please Note: The information contained in this Hormone Balance Test is not intended to replace a one-to-one relationship with a qualified health care professional, nor is it intended as medical advice. This information is simply a guideline for determining the underlying cause of your symptoms. You are encouraged to make your health care decisions in partnership with a qualified health care professional.

Hormone Quiz Answers

The recommended tests are given for each group. You will need to order a saliva/blood spot testing kit. (This information is included in Appendix B on page 150.)

SYMPTOM GROUP 1

Progesterone deficiency: This is the most common hormone imbalance among women of all ages. You may need to change your diet, get off of synthetic hormones (including birth control pills), and you may need to use some progesterone cream. (This is explained in detail in Dr. John Lee's books, *What Your Doctor May Not Tell You About Menopause* and *What Your Doctor May Not Tell You About Premenopause*).

Suggested Testing: saliva testing for progesterone and estradiol

SYMPTOM GROUP 2

Estrogen deficiency: This hormone imbalance is most common in menopausal women—especially if you are petite and/or slim. You may need to make some special changes to your diet, take some women's herbs or use some bioidentical estrogen (about one-tenth the dose prescribed by most doctors).

Suggested Testing: saliva testing for estradiol.

SYMPTOM GROUP 3

Excess estrogen: In women, this is most often solved by getting off of the conventional synthetic hormones most often prescribed by doctors for menopausal women.

SYMPTOM GROUP 4

Estrogen dominance: This is caused when you don't have enough progesterone to balance the effects of estrogen. Thus, you can have low estrogen, but if you have even lower progesterone, you can have symptoms of estrogen dominance. Many women between the ages of 40 and 50 suffer from estrogen dominance. This topic is covered in much detail in Dr. John Lee's timeless book, *What Your Doctor May Not Tell You about Menopause.*

Suggested Testing: Saliva testing for Hormone Profile I or just test for progesterone and estradiol.

SYMPTOM GROUP 5

Excess androgens (male hormones): This is most often caused by too much sugar and simple carbohydrates in the diet and is often found in women who have polycystic ovary syndrome (PCOS). You can find out more about PCOS in *What Your Doctor May Not Tell You About Premenopause.*

Suggested Testing: saliva hormone testing for progesterone, estradiol, testosterone and androstenedione.

SYMPTOM GROUP 6

Cortisol deficiency: This is caused by tired adrenals, which is usually caused by chronic stress. If you're trying to juggle a job and a family, chances are good you have tired adrenals. There are great chapters on restoring your adrenal function in both of Dr. John Lee's books on menopause and premenopause.

Suggested Testing: saliva hormone testing for the adrenal function or one of the individual cortisol tests.

If You Are Still Confused, Try the Following Guidelines:

• If you haven't had a saliva hormone level test before or if you fit into more than one category above, it is ideal if you get "The Works," i.e. Hormone Profile III, to give you the big picture. This is a great way to get baseline measurements of your hormones, *and* it is a very informative and comprehensive analysis.

• If you fit into more than one category above, *including fatigue*, and if you are on a budget, you'll get a lot of useful information from Hormone Profile II.

• If you fit into more than one category *not* including fatigue, try Hormone Profile I.

• If you are primarily having issues with stress and fatigue, try the Adrenal Function or one of the individual cortisol tests.

• If you just want the basics, test for progesterone, estradiol, and testosterone.

• If you have estrogen dominance symptoms and want just a bare bones look at your hormones, just test progesterone and estradiol.

• If you recently started supplementing with progesterone and only want to find out whether your levels are within "normal" ranges, just test progesterone.

• If you have polycystic ovary syndrome (PCOS) and/or symptoms of excess male hormones such as excess hair growth, test progesterone, estradiol, testosterone and androstenedione.

• If you have PMS, endometriosis, infertility or postpartum blues, you'll get a lot of helpful information listed in the testing kit instructions.

Once you have had the testing done and realize the need for some type of hormone replacement, it is important to follow careful guidelines regarding that replacement. In her book *The Schwarzbein Principle: The Program*, Dr. Diana Schwarzbein gives four basic rules for hormone replacement:

1. **Identify the hormone(s) that need to be replaced.** Although you do not have to wait for a hormone to be completely gone before starting to replace it, do not replace a hormone that can still be produced appropriately. Laboratory work is the best way to identify missing hormones. Unfortunately, not all labs can run hormone levels accurately; therefore, your blood or saliva samples need to be run through specific labs. (Check for specific recommendations in Appendix B on page 150 or go to Dr. Diana Schwarzbein's Web site at *www.schwarzbeinprinciple.com*).

2. **Replace the missing hormone with the same (identical) hormone.** Bioidentical hormones are the same in chemical structure as the hormones your body makes whether they are found in nature or made in a lab (synthetic). Everything else is a drug to your body and, therefore, toxic. Never take drug hormones instead of bioidentical ones. Premarin is a drug estrogen while estradiol preparation is bioidentical to estradiol (the human estrogen made in the ovaries). Do not confuse hormones found in nature with natural hormones. The term "natural hormones" includes synthetic hormones as long as the synthetic hormone is bioidentical in structure to the one your body used to make. For example, the T4

> **Researchers to Supervisory Panel:**
>
> "Our new product has no fat, no cholesterol, no calories, no sugar, no salt, and no preservatives. The box is empty, but it has exactly what everyone wants."

and T3 preparations used in the treatment of hypothyroidism are mostly made in a laboratory, but they are bioidentical in structure to the T4 and T3 found in the human body and therefore are natural hormones. Hence, switching the terminology to bioidentical is less confusing than the word natural. Once you have been given a prescription for a bioidentical hormone, it is time to move on to rule number 3, the hardest component of hormone replacement therapy to accomplish—but one that is achievable.

3.   **Match the replaced hormone's normal**

Ways to Know if You Have "Estrogen Issues":

1.   Everyone around you has an attitude problem.
2.   You add chocolate chips to your cheese omelet.
3.   The dryer has shrunk every last one of your skirts.
4.   Your husband is suddenly agreeing to everything you say.
5.   You're using your cellular phone to dial up every bumper sticker that says "How's my driving, call 1-800-…."
6.   Everyone's head looks like an invitation to batting practice.
7.   You're sure that everyone is scheming to drive you crazy.
8.   The ibuprofen bottle is empty, and you bought it yesterday.

production and secretion. This is difficult and often inconvenient to do. For example, a person who has Type I diabetes needs to take insulin shots. To exactly mimic the way the pancreas makes and secretes insulin is impossible because there are too many variables, so try to match insulin dosing to food intake only. That is good enough—but not perfect—and requires the person with diabetes to take multiple shots of differing amounts of insulin throughout the day. It would be more convenient for this person to take one big shot of insulin a day. However, this will not work because the body does not secrete insulin in one big dose every day. Whatever bioidentical hormone replacement therapy you are taking, try to match the replaced hormone's normal production and secretion for the best results.

4.   **Take hormone replacement therapy seriously.** HRT needs to be tracked with lab tests and physician follow-up visits. This may seem obvious if you have Type I diabetes or thyroid disease, but this rule is usually ignored [when women are going through (or experiencing)] menopause. It is important to follow every parameter available for each hormone deficiency state. With diabetes, this involves the patient's doing home blood-glucose monitoring and then having more intensive lab work and physician follow-up visits on a regular basis. Menopausal women need to have their estradiol and progesterone levels measured by a good lab and reviewed by their

physician. They should also track their withdrawal periods and keep up with breast self-exams, pap smears, bone mineral density studies, and uterine ultrasound evaluations, if indicated.

Infertility: A Common Problem

As a lay person, I am not qualified to adequately teach the entire spectrum of infertility. However, there is one cause of infertility that I want to present in this chapter—a lack of progesterone. A woman may have enough progesterone to get the egg developed and down the fallopian tubes where it may be fertilized but not have enough to keep it on the wall. The ovaries have follicles that are responsible for getting the egg developed. Every month the body wants to do what it was created to do—procreate a human being. However, if there is a lack of progesterone in the body, it is difficult to provide enough progesterone to develop the egg. Because the body tries so hard to develop the egg without the necessary progesterone, "follicle burnout" is the result. The follicles just cannot do it any more. If there is not a structural problem in the body preventing the egg from being developed, there is a high probability that the body has a deficiency of progesterone.

Many women are seeing positive results by going on a regimen of bioidentical progesterone cream for about four months. This does what some refer to as "taking the follicles on vacation." For four months the follicles do not even think of ovulation. They just "bask in the sun." Dr. John

Question:

How many women with PMS does it take to change a light bulb?

Answer:

One. Only ONE!! And do you know WHY it only takes ONE? Because no one else in this house knows HOW to change a light bulb. They don't even know the bulb is BURNED OUT. They would sit in this house in the dark for THREE DAYS before they figured it OUT. And once they figured it out, they wouldn't be able to find the light bulbs despite the fact that they've been in the SAME CUPBOARD for the past SEVENTEEN YEARS. But if they did, by some miracle, actually find the light bulbs, TWO DAYS LATER the chair that they dragged from two rooms over to stand on to change the STUPID light bulb would STILL BE IN THE SAME SPOT!! AND UNDERNEATH IT WOULD BE THE CRUMPLED WRAPPER THE STUPID LIGHT BULBS CAME IN! WHY?! BECAUSE NO ONE IN THIS HOUSE EVER CARRIES OUT THE GARBAGE!! IT'S A WONDER WE HAVEN'T ALL SUFFOCATED FROM THE PILES OF GARBAGE THAT ARE 12 FEET DEEP THROUGHOUT THE ENTIRE HOUSE! IT WOULD TAKE AN ARMY TO CLEAN THIS...I'm sorry...what did you ask me?

Lee suggests that you apply the progesterone cream on days 5 to 26 so your body doesn't even think ovulation and the follicles can heal. After a few months, stop taking the bioidentical progesterone when menstruation begins. Start taking it again each month on days 14 through 28 of your cycle. This procedure has enabled numbers of ladies suffering from infertility to get pregnant.

Just a few months ago I met a beautiful young mother with her adorable 18-month-old daughter. This lady had been suffering from a number of symptoms including obesity, acne, fatigue, and infertility. She implemented the guidelines in this book, including hormone replacement therapy—bioidentical progesterone. She did not look like the same person. She is trim, has lots of energy (needed to keep up with that 18-month-old toddler!), and was able to get pregnant.

For more information on infertility, you will want to read Dr. John Lee's book *What Your Doctor May Not Tell You About Premenopause.*

STEP FIVE PRINCIPLES

1. If, after instituting steps one through four of this unit, you still are not feeling well and seem to have a hormone imbalance, consider bioidentical hormone replacement.

2. Have your hormones tested using saliva and blood spot testing.

3. Labs which process saliva testing are listed in Appendix B on page 150.

4. Once you have received your lab results, have them interpreted by a physician who is able to then prescribe the necessary hormone replacement.

5. If you require some type of hormone replacement, use only bioidentical hormones.

Why God Invented Menopause…

With all the new technology regarding fertility, a 73 year-old woman gave birth to a baby. When she was discharged from the hospital and went home, her relatives came to visit.

"May we see the new baby?" one asked.

"Not yet," said the 73 year-old mother. "Soon."

Thirty minutes had passed, and another relative asked, "May we see the new baby now?"

"Not yet," said the mother.

After another few minutes had elapsed, they asked again, "May we see the baby now?"

"No!" replied the mother.

Growing very impatient, they asked, "Well, when CAN we see the baby?"

"WHEN IT CRIES," she told them.

"WHEN IT CRIES?" they demanded. "Why do we have to wait until it CRIES?"

"BECAUSE, I forgot where I put it…"

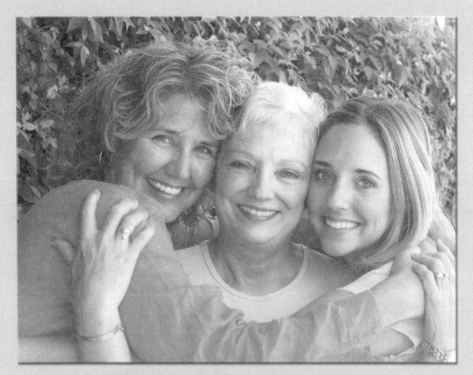

PART FIVE

Obesity and Poor Health:
A Struggle or a Stronghold?

Struggle or Stronghold?

One of the more obvious symptoms of poor health in women is obesity. Now, clearly, that is not the only symptom, but it does seem to be one of the most common. For many women, weight gain and/or poor health is something that began in their late thirties or early forties. They have been temperate in their eating all of their adult lives and have worked to keep their weight in check. For these ladies, the problem is usually not out-of-control eating, but a hormone imbalance that has occurred as they are entering the menopausal years.

However, for ladies who have struggled with obesity for years (and intermittently won the battle for brief periods of time in their adult lives only to eventually return to old habits), the obesity is often a sign of a more serious problem—a spiritual stronghold in one's life. Mrs. Frieda Cowling has written an excellent book entitled *Principles of Weight Control.* Frieda (who wears the same size dress she wore when she was married) says that her rules have worked for her for 40 years, and she weighs 125 pounds at age 65! She says,

Keeping my weight under control is a battle I will fight for the rest of my life. It will never be easy for me because I love eating and am a glutton. The older I get, the harder I struggle to follow my rules; but I refuse to be defeated. If I can keep my weight down, so can you![1]

I agree with Frieda 100 percent! However, for many people who have not kept their weight in check their entire adult lives as Frieda Cowling has, weight control has become more than a struggle; it has become a stronghold. II Corinthians 10:3–5 says, *"For though we walk in the flesh, we do not war after the flesh: (For the weapons of our warfare are not carnal, but mighty through God to the pulling down of strong holds;) Casting down imaginations, and every high thing that exalteth itself against the knowledge of God, and bringing into captivity every thought to the obedi-*

> From "Men's Rules for Women":
>
> "If you think you're fat, you probably are. Don't ask us. We refuse to answer."

ence of Christ." What is a stronghold? Dr. Jack Schaap has written a book on unclean spirits and goes into detail about strongholds in our lives. He says, "A stronghold is a fortress shrine for evil spirits."[2]

Once that fortress is built, it is not easily torn down. Unclean spirits gain entrance into our lives through the works of the flesh which are listed in Galatians 5:17-21. For this reason Titus 2:12 admonishes us, *"Teaching us that, denying ungodliness and worldly lusts, we should live soberly, righteously, and godly, in this present world…."* Allowing unclean spirits to work with our flesh in setting up strongholds in our lives is inviting the enemy to come and live within. There is no way we can live the victorious Christian life that Jesus intended if we are entertaining the enemy within through our besetting sins. Rather than living a life for God, we are actually allowing ourselves to become His enemy. James 4:4b says, *"…whosoever therefore will be a friend of the world is the enemy of God."*

Signs That You Might Be Experiencing Menopause…

- You sell your home heating system at a yard sale.
- Your husband jokes that instead of buying a wood stove, he is using you to heat the family room this winter.
- You write post-it notes with your kids' names on them.
- You change your underwear after every sneeze.

My entire adult life I have had to work at weight control. It has always been interesting to me that when I controlled what I ate, I had victory in other areas of my life, and my entire life was so much more in order. In my late twenties I had become quite undisciplined in my eating habits and went to a dear friend and co-worker for help. She did help me tremendously by giving me Biblical principles by which to live. In the process I lost weight and had a more structured and orderly lifestyle. It was at that same time that I also instituted some procedures to help me have a more faithful walk with God. I did not have the knowledge and understanding at the time to realize that the steps I took actually helped to tear down a stronghold of gluttony in my life.

After my daughter Carissa was born, I was able to control my weight until I quit nursing. At that time I began putting on a little bit of weight. I'm sure the hormonal changes in my body contributed in part to some of weight gain, but I know that I also returned to some out-of-control eating habits and thus unknowingly invited those unclean spirits back which had been knocked out of my life several years prior.

When Carissa was about two years of age, I talked with a good friend of mine and told her my frustration about my weight. She agreed to be of help to me, but she gave me some conditions and guidelines (Biblical principles) she expected of me. I began instituting those guidelines, but my flesh rebelled. I clearly recall after a few weeks of struggle the day I thought, "This fight is just too hard. It's just not worth all the hassle." I called my friend and told her that it just "wouldn't work" for me to work with her on my weight control.

I believe with all of my heart that the choice I made that day would wreak havoc in my life for many years. I had no idea at the time that I was saying to those unclean spirits who had been invited back into my life by my out-of-control appetites, "You know what? It's too hard to clean you out. You can just stay put." When I stated at the beginning of the book that I have no one to blame but me for my years of poor health, I meant it. I believe that I struggled for years because I did not get to the root problem—a stronghold that was set up in my life.

It seemed that no matter how I tried to lose weight, I could not do it. Nor could I seem to find help for my poor health. I do not believe that God was being mean to me; I believe He wanted me to do more than just lose weight. He wanted me to get rid of a very big stronghold in my life. My road to regaining my health started when I went to God and began *begging* for His help.

I did not realize for a number of years that my battle for good health and proper weight control was also truly a battle over a stronghold in my life. I did realize that it was not just a physical battle but also a spiritual battle. I did not realize that at the root of my struggles was a stronghold that the Devil and his dirty imps did not want to give up. In the past few years, especially through the preaching and teaching of my pastor, God has given me a new understanding of strongholds, the havoc they wreak in our lives (and the lives of those around us), and the process involved in gaining victory over those strongholds. I also understand that any time I give up the daily fight and give in to out-of-control appetites, the unclean spirits will come back in and defile my life!

Please know that I am not stating that all overweight people have a stronghold of gluttony in their lives. Sometimes obesity is simply a result of a hormonal imbalance and a damaged metabolism. I have seen numbers of ladies who could not understand why they were having weight-control issues or health problems when they reached their late thirties or forties. The ladies had been temperate in their eating habits and had been effective in their weight control and had felt well for years. When these ladies have instituted the principles outlined in Part Four, they have seen immediate results and have been able to get back on track. I do not believe every woman who is struggling with her health and/or weight control has a stronghold of gluttony.

I do, however, believe that I had that problem, and I have talked with a number of ladies who also struggle with strong-

> ## Two Cats Talking:
> "Having nine lives is great, but if I have to go through menopause again, forget it!

holds that are preventing good health and effective weight control. If you have come to realize that a big part of your problem with poor health and effective weight control is due, in a large part, to a spiritual stronghold in your life, you will be helped by the principles I give in this chapter and in the other recommended reading I suggest.

I would like to emphasize that it is not just the eating aspect of women's health that can be a stronghold. I have talked with a small percentage of very trim ladies who are in poor health who don't seem to really want answers. It almost appears that their poor health is an addiction of sorts. I can never judge other women or decide who has what type of stronghold in her life, but I have talked with ladies who make statements that seem to indicate that they like the attention they receive over their poor health more than they want good health. Other ladies seem to almost get a "high" from being a martyr, doing the Lord's work to the detriment of their health as they brag about how sick they are or how tired they are as they've worked late into the night on projects or gone days without proper rest or proper food. Some ladies tell all about their poor health but laugh off real answers with statements such as, "Yes, my husband tells me I need to do that, too!"

> PMS really stands for "Purchase More Shoes."

These ladies are addicted to the synthetic "highs" they receive as a result of their poor health.

I believe most of us

don't realize just how serious it is when we keep a stronghold in our lives. Numbers of ladies want to be thin, to be in good health, and to feel good, but the stronghold that plagues them sometimes has such a grasp on their lives that they would rather keep the stronghold than have the victory.

Xenocomforters

Many ladies do not face poor health issues alone; they also face the fact that the abusive lifestyle that has caused the poor health is a stronghold in their lives. If this is your situation, it is important to realize that the Devil does not give in easily in these situations. That stronghold is a "trophy" of what he can do in the Christian's life, so he does not want to give it up.

In chapter thirteen I explained "xenoestrogens." These are imitation estrogens. They are not the real thing, but they do look and act like the real thing. The Devil is the master imitator! For every real thing God provides, the Devil has come up with an imitation. I believe in the area of besetting sins and strongholds, the Devil has devised an imitation comforter—a *xenocomforter* if you will.

Before Jesus ascended to Heaven after His resurrection from the dead, He talked with His disciples and gave some instruction and some words of encouragement. John 14:16–18a says, *"And I will pray the Father, and he shall give you another Comforter, that he may abide with you for ever; Even the Spirit of truth; whom the world cannot* receive, *because it seeth him not, neither knoweth him: but ye know him; for he dwelleth with you, and shall be in you. I will not leave you comfortless...."*

Jesus knew the difficulties and the trials that Christians would face through the centuries, so He said, "Hey, guys, I'm going on to Heaven, but don't worry. I'm going to send Someone else to comfort you when you go through the hard times. That Comforter is the Holy Spirit."

The Devil heard this and said, "Oh, man, I can't let that happen. I've got to have a substitute comfort for these Christians. So, he devised "besetting sins." The Devil offers synthetic comforters for us to turn to during times of trial and stress. Pastor Jack Schaap defines besetting sins as "those sins where we turn for comfort." The problem with the Devil's *xenocomforters* is that they are addicting. Therefore, these besetting sins become strongholds in our lives, and they are where we turn for comfort instead of to the "REAL" source of comfort, the Holy Spirit.

I have never enjoyed poor health. I have never enjoyed the pain, the foggy thinking, the fatigue, the obesity, etc., but I did enjoy eating the wrong foods (and still have the desire, I might add!) One of the reasons that regaining my health has been a long process is that I did enjoy eating the wrong foods. That desire for wrong foods was a stronghold in my life. I would eat right for a season but then get tired of the fight and return to my old ways.

I love to eat. I am a glutton as much as (or probably more than) Frieda Cowling is. But there came a day in my life when I realized I was putting great limitations on being used of God as I held on to my stronghold. There came a day when I decided that I wanted victory in my life more than I wanted that stronghold. I wanted the abundant life more than I wanted the stronghold. As I have gotten a vision of the Judgment Seat of Christ, I have wanted to get rid of that stronghold in order to do all I can do for God in my lifetime.

Strongholds Limit My Work for God

Second Corinthians 5:10 says, *For we must all appear before the judgment seat of Christ; that every one may receive the things done in his body, according*

Skip-a-Day Diet Plan:

Mrs. Lee was terribly overweight, so her doctor put her on a diet. "I want you to eat regularly for two days, then skip a day, and repeat this procedure for two weeks. The next time I see you, you'll have lost at least five pounds."

When Mrs. Lee returned, she shocked the doctor by losing nearly 20 pounds. "Why, that's amazing!" the doctor said. "Did you follow my instructions?"

Mrs. Lee nodded. "I'll tell you, though, I thought I was going to drop dead that third day."

"From hunger, you mean?" the doctor asked.

"No, from skipping," she answered.

to that he hath done, whether it be good or bad." We do have a very loving God, but He is also a God Who expects us to do more than lie around and eat bonbons all day! God left us on this earth to do a work for Him; one day we will give account of this life. He gave up His Son Jesus Christ Who came to this earth and lived a sinless life for 33 years only to be crucified by an angry mob. I do not begin to understand Calvary, but I do know that in His death, burial, and resurrection Jesus suffered my hell for me. I can't comprehend it, but Jesus suffered the eternal punishment for every sinner when He died on the cross. What a great Saviour! What a debt I owe a God Who gave His all to rescue me from spending an eternity in Hell!

At the Judgment Seat of Christ I will receive rewards for every work I have done for eternity. First Corinthians 3:12–15 says, *"Now if any man*

You Know You Are Addicted to Coffee if…

* You grind your coffee beans in your mouth.
* You sleep with your eyes open.
* You can jumpstart your car without cables.
* You walk 20 miles on your treadmill before you realize it's not plugged in.
* You short out motion detectors.
* You soak your dentures in coffee overnight.

build upon this foundation gold, silver, precious stones, wood, hay, stubble; Every man's work shall be made manifest: for the day shall declare it, because it shall be revealed by fire; and the fire shall try every man's work of what sort it is. If any man's work abide which he hath built thereupon, he shall receive a reward. If any man's work shall be burned, he shall suffer loss: but he himself shall be saved; yet so as by fire." I don't want to stand before Christ empty handed; I want it to be very evident at the judgment seat of Christ that my life proved my gratitude, love, and adoration to a great God and Saviour! (And besides, I really do like "gold, silver, and precious stones!")

God wants clean vessels to use for His work, but allowing a stronghold to remain "dirties up" my vessel. When my daughter Carissa was growing up, she had the responsibility of making sure the dishwasher got turned on when it was full. We are a family of three, so usually putting in the dirty dishes from one meal does not fill the dishwasher. One summer when she had gone to church camp, I started to set the table for dinner. I opened the cupboards to get dishes and found the cupboards empty—no glasses, no plates, and no silverware. I opened the dishwasher and began removing dishes thinking I would just use the clean ones from the dishwasher. I was quite surprised to find dirty dishes but then realized that Carissa was not home. I had been putting dirty dishes in and had failed to turn on the dishwasher! Now, I did not use those dishes as they were; I washed them in the sink (the old-fashioned way like I did when I was growing up!).

Did I have it in for those dirty dishes? NO! Did I think I was better than those dirty dishes? NO! Was the problem that those dishes were not as good as new ones I could get at the store? NO! I just don't particularly like to eat off of dirty dishes! When I keep sin in my life, God's reason for not using me in ways He would like to for eternity is not because He has it in for me. He simply does not use dirty vessels for His work any more than I use dirty dishes when I serve food to my family! If I am going to do all I can for eternity and thoroughly enjoy the Judgment Seat of Christ, I must be a clean vessel! In order to be a clean vessel, I must get rid of strongholds in my life.

Strongholds Affect Future Generations

A second reason I became determined to get rid of the strongholds in my life is that they so affect future generations. Deuteronomy 5:9 and Exodus 20:5 both say, *"Thou shalt not bow down thyself unto them, nor serve them: for I the LORD thy God am a jealous God, visiting the iniquity of the fathers upon the children unto the third and fourth generation of them that hate me."* Numbers 14:18 says, *"The LORD is longsuffering, and of great mercy, forgiving iniquity and transgression, and by no means clearing the guilty, visiting the iniquity of the fathers upon the children unto the third and fourth generation."* God only needs to say something once for

us to realize that is what He believes about that particular subject. When He repeats something three times, He's putting emphasis on that truth to make a powerful statement to us. He is warning me that the sins I hold onto in my life and the strongholds I keep are going to affect my daughter Carissa and her children and their children!

I love my daughter too much to hang on to my strongholds and allow them to be passed down to the next generation! I don't want my grandchildren to have to look back at their grandmother and think, "You know, she had a problem with food, she never got victory, and she has passed that stronghold on to me!" Proverbs 13:22 says, *"A good man leaveth an inheritance to his children's children: and the wealth of the sinner is laid up for the just."* If I'm going to leave an inheritance to my grandchildren, I want it to be a good inheritance, not the inheritance of a spiritual stronghold like an addiction to wrong foods!

Our pastor says that problems are both practical and spiritual in nature. There are a number of practical steps I've had to take to regain my

Thyroid Testing:

Mrs. Smith was having difficulty in losing some added pounds she had acquired in recent months. However, the doctor smirked when Mrs. Smith requested that he run a thyroid test to see if her problem could be hypothyroidism. Evidently he smelled the chocolate chip cookies on her breath!

health, but if I only address the practical (the five basic principles I gave in Part Four to regain one's health), then I have only given part of the solution. We must also address the spiritual. Wrong habits—whether it is eating wrong food, not properly dealing with stress, or not getting enough rest are both a spiritual and a practical problem; therefore, the problem must be addressed on both a practical and a spiritual level.

Take a look at your life. Are there strongholds you have that are part of the problem related to your health? Do you seem unable to get victory in your eating habits and in your health-related lifestyle? If so, decide today that you are going to take the necessary steps to pull down the strongholds and get the complete victory God so desperately wants you to have!

Bumper Sticker:

"I'm out of estrogen, and I've got a gun."

Tearing Down the Stronghold

One way I feel very loved by God is the fact that He gives me answers—real solutions—to problems I am facing. Answers to tearing down the strongholds in my life came in steps, not all at once. I would like to share the process I experienced.

"Lord, Be Thorough with Me!"

The first step for me came from a sermon Dr. Jack Schaap preached just a few months after he became pastor of First Baptist Church of Hammond, Indiana. He told the story of the great evangelist Curtis Hutson who had died of cancer in March of 1995. Dr. Hutson came to a point in his life where he felt he was not doing all he could do for God. He felt there were things in his life that were limiting God from using him, so he began praying, "Lord, be thorough with me."

When I first heard that illustration, I was convicted, but I did not want to begin praying that prayer. Curtis Hutson had died of cancer, and I didn't want to get cancer as a result of my praying, "Lord, be thorough with me."

However, after a few weeks I realized that I could get cancer and die whether I prayed that prayer or not. My praying that prayer did not mean I would get cancer any more than not praying it would prevent my getting cancer. And so, I began to daily pray, "Lord, be thorough with me." That was five years ago. I wish I could tell you all of the blessings that have come to my life as a result.

I do get the sense that God is being thorough with me. The Christian life is a journey, not a destination. I will never "arrive" at perfection and complete victory in this lifetime. God did not just do one big "whiz-bang" job and say, "There! I've been thorough with you, and you are all fixed up." When I began praying, I said, "Now, Lord, You know how much I can take without getting discouraged and turning back. I want You to be as thorough with me as I can handle at a time."

Probably I could have learned and grown more quickly, but I have had the sense that God has been patient with me these past five years. I haven't always liked what He was doing, but I have always liked the end result as He has helped me to grow.

I have seen God do a work to clean up an

area in my life and follow that correction with a special opportunity to serve Him. Let me illustrate. For several years I'd had the dream to teach an adult ladies' Sunday school class. One year to the week after I began praying for God to be thorough with me, Pastor Schaap called me and asked me to teach an adult ladies' Sunday school class. Weekly as I teach the Friendship Class, I am reminded that I asked God to be thorough with me, and He heard my prayer. I believe that had I refused to invite God into my life to do the work that He wanted to do, I would not be teaching that Sunday school class. That is just one illustration of many I could give. Trust me. You will never regret—especially at the Judgment Seat of Christ—asking God to be thorough with you and to do a cleansing work in your life! Again, it won't always be pleasant, and it won't be easy, but oh, it's so worth it!

I believe that we fail to realize how many opportunities we miss because we don't allow God to clean us up. We are comfortable with our sin, and the thought of having to give up some things or change some habits does not appeal to our flesh. Had I refused to submit to God's correction, I believe I would have wondered why He never gave me the opportunity to teach an adult ladies' Sunday school class, nor would I have realized that God withheld that opportunity because of my hardheartedness! Do today what you know you should do, and you'll be glad at the Judgment Seat of Christ!

A Change of Mind

A second step toward victory came in the form of an article in the *Christian Womanhood* magazine. I have found that because of strongholds in my life, implementing the proper principles for good health has not been easy. Strongholds don't go away easily; they must be cast down. One month in *Christian Womanhood*, Mrs. Schaap discussed a stronghold she had to deal with in her own life. She made some statements in that article that God used to change my life:

> Before my life could be changed, my mind had to be changed, which is true for every Christian…In spite of a season of depression, I continued to seek the Word of God more diligently than ever and resisted the desire to try some other "fix." The Word of God does work; it is the answer…for everything!…One day God took His strong hand and pushed away all the bricks of 'stinking thinking' that were stacking in my mind. It seemed that I took two steps forward and then one step back; yet, in a way it seems that He did it all at once…God is the Almighty, and He does have the power to change your life and your mind.[1]

Her article helped me to put a label on my struggle—"stronghold." Her words made me realize more than ever that one of the great ingredients to victory is the Word of God! Hence, I intensified my Bible reading, memory, and meditation. The Word of God is a powerful Book and a required tool in tearing down our strongholds. Hebrews 4:12 says, *"For the word of God is quick, and powerful, and sharper than any twoedged sword, piercing even to the dividing asunder of soul and spirit, and of the joints and marrow, and is a discerner of the thoughts and intents of the heart."* II Timothy 3:16 says, *"All scripture is given by inspiration of God, and is profitable for doctrine, for reproof, for correction, for instruction in righteousness."* Our thinking needs to be corrected, and the Word of God is the Source of that correction.

Other verses that reveal our great need to fill our minds with the Word of God include I Corinthians 2:16: *"For who hath known the mind of the Lord, that he may instruct him? But we have the mind of Christ."* (which is the Word of God) and Philippians 2:5: *"Let this mind be in you, which was also in Christ Jesus."*

Tearing Down the Strongholds

God used Mrs. Schaap's article to take me to a new level of victory, but I still needed more work done to tear down the stronghold of my addiction to wrong food. God sweetly gave me more help through a Wednesday night Bible study series our pastor taught on unclean spirits in our lives. Pastor Schaap spent a number of weeks explaining unclean spirits in our lives and the strongholds they build. That Bible study gave me

a new understanding of the battle I was fighting. In order to win the victory, it is very important to understand just who you are fighting and how the enemy works. The battle we are fighting is a spiritual battle with the Devil and his army of dirty little imps!

I was thrilled when Pastor Schaap chose to compile those Bible studies into a book entitled, *Opening the Door to the Unclean Spirits.* I believe that it is imperative for **anyone** who is struggling with strongholds to get that book and read it. *(You may purchase that book from Christian Womanhood by going to www.christianwomanhood.org or by calling (219) 365-3202. The cost at the time of this writing is $15 plus shipping and handling.)* If your struggle with poor health and proper weight control is because of a spiritual stronghold, I believe the teaching of Pastor Schaap's book is more important than the practical principles I will be giving you in the last section of this book. Don't get me wrong, the principles I am giving you work and will help you regain your health, but the number-one key for those whose ill health is a result of a spiritual stronghold would be to order that book today and study it at the same time you are reading and studying this book.

Strongholds are established in our lives through a process. Pastor Schaap explains,

First, the Christian committed a fleshly sin. Second, the fleshly sin brought in a filthy spirit. Third, the filthy spirit brought in other unsavory fellows. Last, the unsavory fellows banded together and built a castle or stronghold in the Christian's life. Building a stronghold is the ultimate goal for unclean spirits. Why? A castle does two things for these spirits. It ensures their longevity in the life of the Christian, and it honors their master…A stronghold in the life of a Christian is a special trophy to Satan. It is more of a credit to Satan's abilities to set up a shrine there than it is in the heart of an unbeliever.[2]

The reason getting rid of these strongholds in our lives is so difficult is that Satan and his demons are not going to give up their real estate without a fight. They work hard to keep it. For that reason, once a Christian decides he is going to get rid of that stronghold, the Devil sends reinforcements to keep his territory. That is why things usually get worse before they get better!

But God is a great and mighty God Who wants us to have victory and has provided the path for victory. Notice the process in II Corinthians 10:3-6: *"For though we walk in the flesh, we do not war after the flesh: (For the weapons of our warfare are not carnal, but mighty through God to the pulling down of strong holds;) Casting down imaginations and every high thing that exalteth itself against the knowledge of God, and bringing into captivity every thought to the obedience of Christ; And having in a readiness to revenge all disobedience, when your obedience is fulfilled."*

1.   Realize that this is a spiritual battle, not a fleshly battle. That is why five basic principles to good health are not the total solution for those struggling with poor health. We must have God very involved to win the victory, and we must use His weapons! Those weapons are described in Ephesians 6:11-18: *"Put on the whole armour of God, that ye may be able to stand against the wiles of the devil. For we wrestle not against flesh and blood, but against principalities, against powers, against the rulers of the darkness of this world, against spiritual wickedness in high places. Wherefore take unto you the whole armour of God, that ye may be able to withstand in the evil day, and having done all, to stand. Stand therefore, having your loins girt about with truth, and having on the breastplate of righteousness; And your feet shod with the preparation of the gospel of peace; Above all, taking the shield of faith, wherewith ye shall be able to quench all the fiery darts of the wicked. And take the helmet of salvation, and the sword of the Spirit, which is the word of God: Praying always with all prayer and supplication in the Spirit, and watching thereunto with all perseverance and supplication for all saints."* Take note of each piece of armor God has provided so we can win the battle. Then use them!

2.   Get rid of everything that is supporting your stronghold lifestyle. I could have jars and jars of olives in my home and never be tempted to open them. I like olives on a few foods such as Mexican dishes, but I'm not an olive lover. (My dad used to say that he would try an olive every year at Christmas until he learned to like them!

I'm in the boat with him.) However, place some chocolate in my home and I'll find it! My grandmother used to say that somehow I have a sixth sense that can always help me find the chocolate if there is some to be found! Because I really really like chocolate, I don't keep it in my home. There are foods that just don't tempt me much. Potato chips or salty types of crackers are not my downfall, but I could eat several bowls of quality ice cream in an evening! I work hard to keep foods out of my house that will tempt me. I know I cannot have victory without removing the temptation.

3. Have a Spirit-controlled thought life. If I think on some Cold Stone Creamery ice cream long enough, I'll figure out a way to justify a trip to Cold Stone! ("My husband would enjoy this, so I'll take it home for him," or any other number of flimsy excuses will work.) We are given guidelines for proper thinking in Philippians 4:8, *"Finally, brethren, whatsoever things are true, whatsoever things are honest, whatsoever things are just, whatsoever things are pure, whatsoever things are lovely, whatsoever things are of good report; if there be any virtue, and if there be any praise, think on these things."* It is vital to fill our minds with the right thoughts if we are going to have victory!

One of the biggest hurdles we face in gaining victory is the battle in our minds. Right thinking produces right living, and wrong thinking produces wrong living. Proverbs 23:7a says, *"For as he thinketh in his heart, so is he….."* There is a very predictable pattern to our eating wrong foods or violating some other principle of good health. (The Devil has no new tricks!) We tell ourselves why we deserve to eat a particular food—we've been good, we've had a bad day, this little bit of "cheating" won't hurt, or any number of other excuses. All of this "talk" is simply the Devil trying to get us to buy into his lies and defeat us in our quest for a disciplined lifestyle. *Our mind is the battlefield in which our successes and failures are determined by the decisions we make.*

We must realize that in order to change our behavior, we must first change our thinking. Our change in thinking will be effective only to the degree that our thinking becomes the mind of Christ.

• Our thinking is tainted by our sin nature. Isaiah 55:8, 9 says, *"For my thoughts are not your thoughts, neither are your ways my ways, saith the LORD. For as the heavens are higher than the earth, so are my ways higher than your ways, and my thoughts than your thoughts."* I pray nearly every day, "Lord, help me learn Your thoughts and Your ways today."

• Any thinking that is not in line with the Word of God is pride and sin. When we choose our own thoughts and ways above the thoughts and ways of God, we are exalting ourselves above God and His Word! The Bible says in Psalm 10:4, *"The wicked, through the pride of his countenance, will not seek after God: God is not in all his thoughts."*

• Confess and forsake the sin of wrong thinking in order to have victory. James 5:16 says, *"Confess your faults one to another, and pray one for another, that ye may be healed. The effectual fervent prayer of a righteous man availeth much."* In her book, *Principles of Weight Control,* Frieda Cowling writes several times, "I am a glutton." Now, I just don't think of Frieda as a glutton, but the fact that she has been able to admit that is a key to the victory she has experienced. None of us likes to tell our faults, but we will never have victory until we are able to admit who and what we are in God's eyes. James 5:16 gives two important principles in getting victory over a particular sin—confessing our faults (sins) and praying for each other. I join Frieda Cowling in admitting, "I am a glutton." I also pray for you daily for victory in your struggle.

Proverbs 23:21 says, *"For the drunkard and the glutton shall come to poverty: and drowsiness shall clothe a man with rags."* I'm afraid that too often gluttony is not addressed among Christians for the sin that it is. God puts gluttons (those people who give in to their out-of-control appetites for food) in the same category as drunkards. An important part of confessing sin is first realizing what the sin is and then categorizing it as such. Gluttony is sin!

• Having the mind of Christ is a command. Philippians 2:5 says, *"Let this mind be in you, which was also in Christ Jesus…."* First Corinthians 2:16 says, *"For who hath known the mind of the Lord,*

that he may instruct him? But we have the mind of Christ." Of course, the mind of Christ is the Word of God. Our greatest weapon is the Word of God. It is the Word of God that is going to change our thinking and, consequently, our behavior.

Therefore, let me urge you to join me in doing the following:

1. Read the Word of God daily. Read, read, read. Keep a Bible with you and read a chapter or a portion of a chapter when you are waiting or have a few extra minutes. Read the Word of God.

2. Memorize the Word of God. Write the passage you are memorizing on a 3x5 card and keep it with you. Work on memorizing it throughout the day. Go to sleep at night quoting what you have memorized.

3. Listen to the preaching of the Word of God. We have a wonderful resource in men of God preaching the Word of God. Of course, faithfulness to all church services is a given, but also, keep CDs with you and listen to them as you clean your house, as you drive, or as you do any other task. There are also now a number of Internet sites that have Internet radio and offer great preaching by Fundamental Baptist preachers. I often go online to the Webcast at www.fbchammond.com to hear preaching. It is uplifting, inspiring, and helps me live in victory.

Exalt the Word of God in your life to get God's thoughts—to learn and implement the mind of Christ.

4. Implicitly obey the Word of God. I'll be honest, I don't like every command in the Bible. There are times on Saturday mornings when I wish I was not commanded to go soul winning. I'd like to sleep later or spend my Saturday doing things I want to do, but if I'm going to have victory over my stronghold, I must obey and go soul winning! I don't always want to tithe, but that 10 percent of all my increase belongs to God. If I am going to have victory over my stronghold, I must tithe. I don't always want to get out of bed in the morning and spend time in prayer, but if I'm going to have victory over my stronghold, I must get up and pray every day. If I am to have victory over my stronghold, I must obey! Dr. Schaap says,

> "...there is only one hope for the Christian who has strongholds in his life—the power of God. When a Christian repeatedly unleashes that power through obedience, unclean spirits will eventually flee."[3]

5. Control your tongue. James 3:2 says, *"For in many things we offend all. If any man offend not in word, the same is a perfect man, and able also to bridle the whole body."*

I used to wonder how in the world controlling my tongue could help me lose weight or have victory in any other area of my life. However, Dr. Schaap's Bible study on breaking down the strongholds in our lives helped to give me the understanding that I needed.

One of the key reasons that unclean spirits gain a stronghold into our lives is that we have out-of-control tongues. An out-of-control tongue advertises to unclean spirits that they are welcome in our lives. However, it is not just the words that we speak with our tongues that get us into trouble. The words we speak come from the thoughts we think. Matthew 12:34b says, *"...for out of the abundance of the heart the mouth speaketh."*

If you want victory over a stronghold in your life, it is vital that your thought life and the words you speak are in accordance with Philippians 4:8 which says, *"Finally, brethren, whatsoever things are true, whatsoever things are honest, whatsoever things are just, whatsoever things are pure, whatsoever things are lovely, whatsoever things are of good report; if there be any virtue, and if there be any praise, think on these things."*

We have a wonderful God Who really does want to tear down those strongholds. Please don't give up. Everyone who makes the decision to get rid of the strongholds in her life will come to a point when it seems too hard. It is at that time she must get reinforcements (extra time in the Word of God, extra prayer time, etc.) in order to have the strength to press on and see the spiritual victory. It is available to all Christians, no matter what the stronghold!

If a stronghold has been built in your life, let me once again urge you to read and study Dr. Jack Schaap's book, *Opening the Door to the*

Unclean Spirits. I have shared some Biblical thoughts and principles in this chapter to help you, but it is too big of a subject to adequately cover in one chapter. Dr. Schaap spent hours studying and preparing the Bible studies he taught and included in his book. You will be blessed, and your life will be transformed if you will make the effort to get his book and incorporate the principles he teaches.

"Lord, Heal My Soul"

Two of the greatest tools God has provided to enable us to see victory in our eating habits are the Word of God and prayer. Life is an exciting journey when we daily implement these tools.

On my daily prayer list, I ask God to help me in my struggle with weight control. I also read, memorize, meditate on, and study the Word of God. As we are faithful in our walk with God, I believe He hears our prayers and gives us special nuggets of truth from His Word.

One day as I was reading Psalm 41, I was intrigued by verse four which says, *"I said, LORD, be merciful unto me: heal my soul; for I have sinned against thee."* I decided to look up the word *heal* in my *Strong's Concordance* which I keep beside my recliner where I read and study my Bible. I was surprised to find that *heal* means "thoroughly repair." I then decided to look up *soul* and was even more surprised to learn that soul refers to "appetites." Of course, included in appetites are a desire for food and drink.

WOW! That was powerful. It gave me a new realization that a struggle with poor health is often a result of broken appetites. Many of us have abused our appetites for years as we have gorged ourselves with wrong foods and perverted our appetites.

As a result of that Bible study, I have added some new words to my daily prayer list—"Dear Lord, heal my soul; Lord, thoroughly repair my appetites." I encourage you to do the same; ask God to heal your appetites in order for your body to be able to heal your metabolism.

I also pray daily that God will tear down my strongholds. I don't trust my flesh. I realize that at any moment my flesh can rear its ugly head and allow unclean spirits to take up residence in my life again. I never want that to happen, so I just keep asking God to tear down the strongholds.

My Opportunity to Please God

Mark 12:41–44 and Luke 21:1–4 tell the story of the widow's mite. Here was a poor widow who had very little of this world's goods. It does not seem fair that she was so poor. It doesn't seem fair that she had to struggle the way she did financially. It just doesn't seem fair that she had such a great lack and such a great struggle. Then, she gave all that she had in the area where she lacked the most. Jesus was impressed! So impressed was He, in fact, that He recorded this woman's deed twice in His Word for all future generations to read.

Why was Jesus so impressed with this woman's exceptionally small gift? I believe one of the great reasons is that though it was small—very, very, very small—it was all that she had, and her giving required great faith. Hebrews 11:6a says, *"But without faith it is impossible to please him...."* Surely the widow's giving of her last mite was a great act of faith as she did not know where her next meal would come from, but she took this step of faith and Jesus noticed. He was pleased!

Have you ever helped in a situation where someone later said, "I couldn't have done that

without you!" You knew that humanly speaking, that was a true statement? It is a great feeling to know that you were so needed and so used. I believe that is how God feels when we let Him know how much we need Him.

So many of us have a "God-is-not-fair" or a "God-has-it-in-for-me" mentality. For a long time I felt it just wasn't fair the way I have struggled all of my adult years with weight control. I felt God was unfair to me in my "lack," and I often complained to Him about His injustice. Why could I not be thin "naturally," or at least have learned the character and principles for proper eating and weight control as a young person? I have also complained to God about the fact that I lose weight so slowly. I wanted the pounds to just "drop off" so I could get on with my life! The fact is, I was mad at God for allowing this struggle in my life.

However, one day I realized that my thinking was very, very wrong. God *is* fair. God is *always* fair, and He is *always* just—*always!* I also realized that my struggle with weight control is my opportunity to give God my "all" in an area where I am so needy. This is my opportunity to go to God and say, "Father, I must have your help. I just can't do this without you." God seemed to say to me, "YES! Those are the words I've been waiting to hear from you!"

Do you feel God has been unfair to you in your struggle with poor health and weight control? Are you angry at God for the struggles you face in controlling your appetites and your weight? I've been there; I've had those attitudes, but let me tell you, those are wasted emotions! This is your opportunity to please God! Step out in faith. Confess your sin of wrong attitudes and give Him your "all"—your attitudes, your weakness, your lack of mind control, your lack of motivation, and your bad habits. Let Him know you just can't do it without Him. Then claim II Corinthians 12:9 which says, *"And he said unto me, My grace is sufficient for thee: for my strength is made perfect in weakness. Most gladly therefore will I rather glory in my infirmities, that the power of Christ may rest upon me."*

Realize that God wants to show Himself strong in the areas where we are the weakest. However, He does have a requirement—our heart must be perfect toward Him. I can't be mad at God and then expect Him to show Himself strong to me. I must realize He is good and He is just, and this is my opportunity to please Him by my faith—only to see Him show Himself strong on my behalf. What a great God we have!!!

Whatever You Do, Don't Give Up!

When I accepted the assignment of being the editor of the women's health column in *Christian Womanhood*, a monthly magazine for Christian ladies, our senior editor, Mrs. Cindy Schaap, said, "Expect some trials; we never take on a new responsibility without the Devil's fighting us." I believed her, but I did not know what to expect. I would find that many of the struggles did not even seem related to weight control.

In January of that year I began a renewed effort of Bible memorization. Many nights I went to sleep reciting in my mind the verses and chapters I had memorized. I also increased the number of preaching tapes I listened to each week. God has used His Word in my life in a great way these past few years. I have continued this practice.

While I have been asking God to be thorough with me and to help me correct those areas that are wrong in my life, I have added to that request. I became very convicted when I read Isaiah 55:8 and 9, *"For my thoughts are not your thoughts, neither are your ways my ways, saith the LORD. For as the heavens are higher than the earth, so are my ways higher than your ways, and my thoughts than your thoughts."* I began praying daily, "Lord, help Your ways and Your thoughts to become my ways and my thoughts."

I have heard it said, "Be careful what you pray; God just may answer you." He has answered my prayer, but I expected Him to "magically" change me. Instead, He sent difficult situations into my life, forcing me to decide how much I really wanted to be like Him.

For example, one day shortly after I began praying for God to help me learn His thoughts and His ways, someone told me another person's opinion about a project on which I was working. I sarcastically answered, "Can I get in the flesh a minute? I really don't give a flip!" I laughed and went on my way. However, minutes later I had this terribly heavy feeling I just couldn't shake. I asked the Holy Spirit what was wrong, and what I had said came to my mind. It was as if God had said to me, "Jane, you say you want My thinking and My ways, but those types of words would never come out of the mouth of Jesus." I called the person and apologized.

Then, someone's words hurt me. Again the

Holy Spirit convicted me, and after work I drove several miles out of my way to go past that person's house to pray for her. I asked God to bless her in a special way that night and to let me know that He had heard me. I was thrilled when I heard the next morning that something really good had happened to her the previous night. God had heard me!

"Now what," you may be asking, "does all of this have to do with breaking down strongholds and getting victory in the area of weight control and good health?" It seems that in my life God connects things. I have seen that the more I try to seek God's mind and His ways (and try to put them into practice), the more strength, wisdom, and discipline He seems to give me in areas where I am struggling.

One of the biggest hurdles I faced was that of not giving up. When something goes slowly, the temptation is to give up. At the time of this writing, I have lost about 30 pounds and gone down two dress sizes! I am grateful that God has given me grace to continue trying to learn proper eating habits rather than giving up. I am not where I want to be, but praise the Lord, neither am I where I used to be. The greatest change, however, is that God is working on me spiritually.

Lest you think that I feel I have arrived, let me assure you that quite the opposite is true.

More than ever I see the holiness of God and the great imperfections and frailties in my own life. We have a wonderfully patient and loving God Who wants to help us. One of my favorite verses that I have claimed many times is II Chronicles 16:9a, *"For the eyes of the LORD run to and fro throughout the whole earth, to shew himself strong in the behalf of them whose heart is perfect toward him…."* He wants to show Himself strong to you, too. He loves you; so do I, and I pray for you daily.

Keep at it. No matter how small your victories, keep on trying. I would also encourage you to begin asking God to teach you His thoughts and His ways. It's a wonderful way to live.

The greatest reason I ask you not to give up, especially if your struggle is a spiritual stronghold, is that the alternative to victory is very depressing. Jesus said in John 10:10, *"The thief cometh not, but for to steal, and to kill, and to destroy: I am come that they might have life, and that they might have it more abundantly."* There is no way to live the abundant life when you allow strongholds to remain in your life. Please note that to allow the stronghold to remain is to let the thief (the Devil and his demons—unclean spirits) to steal, to kill, and to destroy everything that is worthwhile in your life. Please, I beg of you, DON'T GIVE UP!

Afterword

Where Will You Spend Eternity?

I must ask you a most important question before you close the covers of this book. Are you 100 percent sure that you will go to Heaven when you die? I am for everyone's enjoying good health, but if you enjoy good health in this life only, your living is in vain.

Every one of us will die one day. I want to be sure that you are ready to meet the God Who created you. You need to know and understand the following in order to go to Heaven.

- **Realize there is none good.**

Romans 3:10 says, "*As it is written, There is none righteous, no, not one.*"

- **See yourself as a sinner.**

Romans 3:23 says, "*For all have sinned, and come short of the glory of God.*"

- **Recognize where sin came from.**

Romans 5:12 says, "*Wherefore, as by one man sin entered into the world, and death by sin; and so death passed upon all men, for that all have sinned.*"

- **Notice God's price on sin.**

Romans 6:23 says, "*For the wages of sin is death; but the gift of God is eternal life through Jesus Christ our Lord.*"

- **Realize that Christ died for you.**

Romans 5:8 says, "*But God commendeth his love toward us, in that, while we were yet sinners, Christ died for us.*"

- **Take God at His Word.**

Romans 10:13 says, "*For whosoever shall call upon the name of the Lord shall be saved.*"

- **Claim God's promise for your salvation.**

Romans 10:9-11 says, "*That if thou shalt confess with thy mouth the Lord Jesus, and shalt believe in thine heart that God hath raised him from the dead, thou shalt be saved. For with the heart man believeth unto righteousness; and with the mouth confession is made unto salvation. For the scripture saith, Whosoever believeth on him shall not be ashamed.*"

Now pray. Confess that you are a sinner. Ask God to save you and receive Christ as your personal Saviour.

The Four Essential Food Groups

Listed on the following pages you will find lists of each of the food groups containing the foods you should eat in order to have the balanced, nutritional provisions your body needs each day to heal or to maintain a healthy metabolism.

Proteins

Eggs	Soy protein	*Eat Sparingly*	**Nuts & Seeds**
	Tofu	Bleu	*These contain carbohy-*
Beef & Poultry		Brick	*drates so limit intake.*
Beef	**Fish**	Brie	Almonds
Chicken	*Fresh or frozen fish is best;*	Cheddar	Brazil nuts
Duck	*canned or smoked is least*	Colby	Cashews
Lamb	*desirable.*	Edam	Filberts
Pheasant		Gouda	Macadamia nuts
Pork	**Cheese**	Gruyere	Nut butters
Quail	*Best Cheeses to Eat*	Limburger	Peanuts
Turkey	Mozzarella	Monterey Jack	Pecans
Veal	Muenster	Parmesan	Pine nuts
	Neufchatel	Provolone	Pistachio nuts
Soy Products	Ricotta	Romano	Pumpkin seeds
Miso	Queso fresco	Roquefort	Sesame seeds
Tempeh		Swiss	Sunflower seeds
soy milk			Walnuts

- Protein should always be cooked at low, even temperatures.
- Stay away from packaged meats that contain excess salt, sugar, preservatives, and nitrates.
- Everyone needs protein in order to rebuild bones, cells, enzymes, hair, hormones, muscles, nails, and so forth.

Fats

Saturated Fats	Monounsaturated Fats	Polyunsaturated Fats
(To be used for cooking)	*(To be used for cooking)*	*(Not for cooking as these are damaged by heat)*
Butter	Almond oil	
Cheese	Apricot kernel oil	Corn oil
Cream *(Should say "dairy only"—be sure no chemicals are added)*	Avocado oil	Essential fatty acids
	Canola oil	*(Primrose, flaxseed, and borage)*
Nutmeg oil	Grapeseed oil	Salmon oil
Sour cream	Hazelnut oil	Sardine oil
	Olive oil	Sesame seed oil
	Peanut oil	Wheat germ oil

- Our bodies need fats just as they need protein in order to rebuild bones, cells, enzymes, etc.
- Real fats (listed above) are necessary to your body and should be eaten. Do not, however, eat "bad " fats which include: damaged fats (occurs through processing, cooking at high temperatures, or through oxidation—exposure which causes them to become rancid), and man-made fats such as margarine, shortening, imitation sour cream, non-dairy creamers, buttermilk, bottled salad dressings, deep-fried foods, and processed foods.

Nonstarchy Vegetables

Arugula	Cauliflower	Fennel	Kale	Snap beans
Asparagus	Celery	Gardencress	Lettuce	Snow peas
Bamboo shoots	Chayote	Garlic	(not iceberg!)	Shallots
Bean sprouts	Chives	Ginger root	Mushrooms	Spinach
Bell peppers	Collard greens	Green beans	Mustard greens	Summer squash)
Broccoli	Cucumber	Hearts of palm	Onions	Swiss chard
Brussels sprouts	Dandelion greens	Horseradish	Parsley	Tomatoes
Cabbage	Eggplant	Jicama	Peppers	Turnip greens
Carrots	Endive	Jalapeño peppers	Radishes	Watercress

- Nonstarchy vegetables are your body's source of vitamins, minerals, and fiber.
- You may eat as many nonstarchy vegetables as you wish.
- Raw carrots are considered a nonstarchy vegetable; if cooked or juiced, they are considered a carbohydrate.

Carbohydrates

Bread and Crackers
Bread crumbs
Corn tortilla
Cracked-wheat bread
Oat bran bread
Oatmeal bread
Pumpernickel bread
Rice cakes
Rice crackers
Rye crisp bread
Rye wafers
Rye bread
Seven-grain bread
Wheat bran bread
Wheat crackers
Wheat germ bread
Wheat Melba toast
Whole-grain buns
Whole-wheat English muffins
Whole-wheat Matzo
Whole-grain dinner rolls
Whole-grain pita
Whole-grain bread

Fruits
Apples
Applesauce
Apricots
Avocados
Bananas
Blackberries
Blueberries
Boysenberries
Cherries
Crab apples
Cranberries
Currants
Dates
Elderberries
Figs
Gooseberries
Grapefruit
Grapes
Ground cherries
Guavas
Kiwi fruit
Kumquats
Lemons
Limes
Loganberries
Mangos
Melons
Nectarines
Tangerines
Papayas
Passion fruit
Peaches
Pears
Pineapple
Plums
Pomegranate
Prunes
Raisins
Raspberries
Rhubarb
Strawberries
Sun-dried tomatoes
Tomatoes
Tomatillo
Watermelon

Starchy Vegetables
Acorn squash
Artichokes
Beets
Butternut squash
Carrots
Corn
Green peas
Leeks
Lima beans
Okra
Parsnip
Potato
Pumpkin
Rutabagas
Sweet Potato (Yam)
Turnips

Legumes
Adzuki beans
Black beans
Black-eyed peas
Chickpeas
Great Northern beans
Garbanzo beans
Hominy
Kidney beans
Lentils
Mung beans
Navy beans
Pinto beans
Split peas
White beans
Yellow beans

Grains
Barley
Brown rice
Buckwheat
Bulgur
Corn grits
Couscous
Millet
Oats
Polenta
Popcorn
Quinoa
Rye
Semolina
Tapioca
Wheat
Wild rice

Whole-Grain Flour
Amaranth flour
Arrowroot flour
Brown rice flour
Buckwheat flour
Cornmeal
Oat bran flour
Potato flour
Rye flour
Semolina flour
Soy flour
Sunflower seed flour
Whole-wheat flour

- Eating an overabundance of carbohydrates will cause you to gain weight. You need carbohydrates, but in moderation.
- When you consume more carbohydrates than your body needs, the excess will be converted into fats and stored in your fat cells.
- You should always eat carbohydrates with protein and fats.
- It is important to avoid man-made carbohydrates (cakes, candies, ice cream, chips, etc.)
- Do not skip carbohydrates altogether; they are a very needed group of foods in your eating plan.
- Try to eat about 15 grams of carbohydrates per meal.

The possibilities for great meals are almost limitless with such a variety of foods from these four groups! You may read food names with which you are not familiar on these lists. Be brave; branch out and try some new foods. You may want to go to your local library and check out some cookbooks and food-preparation books to learn about these foods and how to prepare and serve them.

Seasonings

Herbs and spices may be used freely in the seasoning of the foods you eat. You may also use the following condiments to season your food: balsamic and other vinegars, fresh garlic, homemade sauces, low-sodium tamari soy sauce, natural mustard, olives, and salsa (made with no sugar added)

Resources

Sources of
Bioidentical Progesterone

If you go to almost any health food store, you will be able to find natural progesterone on the shelves. However, many of these creams do not contain enough progesterone to meet the needs of your body. If the label on the progesterone cream says "wild yam extract," confirm that the product actually contains progesterone and not what companies are calling "precursors" of progesterone such as diosgenin. Also, you want to confirm that the cream contains no petrochemicals (mineral oil, petroleum jelly, and so forth) as these are not only xenoestrogens, they also block absorption into the skin. Listed below is the company where I purchase my progesterone cream.

Arbonne International
Eunice Ray
Phone: 502.241.5552
E-mail: raynation@bluegrass.net

Maker of Prolief and PhytoProlief progesterone creams. This company also provides other non-petrochemical products such as makeup and personal products.

Other sources of natural progesterone cream are listed in Dr. John R. Lee's book, *"What Your Doctor May Not Tell You About Premenopause."*

Salivary Hormone Testing

Aeron Life Cycles
1933 Davis Street, Suite 310
San Leandro, CA 94577
(800) 631-7900

Great Smokies Diagnostic Lab
63 Zilicoa Street
Asheville, NC 28801
(800) 522-4762 (for doctors) or
(888) 891-3061 (for consumers)

David Zava
ZRT Laboratory*
12505 NW Cornell Road
Portland, Oregon 97213
(503) 469-0741
(*This company does occasionally run specials, so you may want to call and ask if they have any current special rates on their testing.)

Resource for Holisitic Physicians

IALP
(800) 927-4227
Ask for the name and phone number of a compounding pharmacy in your area. Once you have the local number, call the pharmacist and ask for the name(s) of any natural or holistic medical doctors in your area.

Recommended Supplements

A word of caution: be aware of the fact that all vitamins are not created equal. Cheap supplements sometimes contain as little as 40 percent or less of the actual vitamin advertised, causing them to be very ineffective. Supplements can be quite expensive, but there are places to get quality products at discounted prices. It is best to purchase pharmaceutical-grade supplements.

Swanson Health Products

(800) 824-4491

Web site: www.swansonvitamins.com

Two recommended brand names from Swanson's are Phytopharmica and Enzymatic Therapy

Puritan's Pride

To order by phone, call (800) 645-1030

Web site: www.puritan.com

Natural Healing and Maintenance Products

Natural Healing Products

Natural Healing Publications

Phone: (877) 832-2463

Web site: www.herbdoc.com

www.womentowomen.com

This is a great Web site to learn more about achieving hormonal balance in the body. There are a lot of practical articles on this Web site to give you a better understanding of how your body works and what it needs to be in hormonal balance.

Oasis Life Sciences

2660 Williamette Drive N.E.

Lacey, WA 98516

Web site: www.lifesciences.com

Following are minimum recommended supplements to take each day:

- Multivitamin and mineral
- Stress B-complex (200 milligrams)
- Omega-3 fatty acids
- Calcium and Magnesium (Take 1,000 milligrams of calcium and half that amount—500 milligrams—of magnesium.)

(Magnesium is a relaxer, so it's best to take magnesium at night. It relaxes you and helps you go to sleep. **Note: If you take thyroid medication, do not take calcium for at least four hours after you have taken your thyroid medication. Calcium will block absorption of the thyroid medication.)**

Additional recommended supplements:
- Potassium
- Vitamin E (200 milligrams)
- Vitamin C (1,000 milligrams)
- Blue-Green Algae (available in capsule or powder form at most health food stores)
- Barley Max (available from Hallelujah Acres, www.hacres.com or (800) 915-9355)

Author's Note: We have made every effort to provide accurate contact information such as phone numbers and Web site addresses. However, this type of information may change after this printing.

Reading Materials for Women's Health

Medical Reference Books on Women's Health

- *Prescription for Nutritional Healing* by James Balch
- *What Your Doctor Might Not Tell You About Menopause* by Dr. John Lee
- *What Your Doctor Might Not Tell You About Premenopause* by Dr. John Lee
- *Healthy Healing* by Linda G. Rector-Page
- *The Schwarzbein Principle* by Diana Schwarzbein
- *The Schwarzbein Principle—The Program* by Diana Schwarzbein [This is the most concise of her books, giving the simplest explanation and principles.]
- *The Schwarzbein Principle II—The Transition* by Diana Schwarzbein
- *The Schwarzbein Principle Cookbook* by Diana Schwarzbein

Christian Reference Books for Stress, Strongholds, and Spiritual Help for Women's Health

The following books are available by contacting Christian Womanhood. To order visit the Web site at www.christianwomanhood.org or call (219) 365-3202.

- *Principles for Proper Weight Control From a Glutton's Point of View* by Frieda Cowling
- *Comfort for Hurting Hearts* by Marlene Evans
- *Living on the Bright Side* by Cindy Schaap
- *Meet the Holy Spirit* by Dr. Jack Hyles
- *Healing for the Inner Hurts* by Dr. Jack Schaap
- *Opening the Door to the Unclean Spirits* by Dr Jack Schaap
- *Walking Through the Valley of Depression and Grief* by Dr. Jack Schaap

Tips for Taking
Bioidentical Progesterone Cream

- **Premenopausal** women should apply one pump of the cream on days 12–26 of their cycle, day one being the first day of your period. **Menopausal** women who are not on any estrogen should apply one pump (preferably at night) for 25 days and then stop for 3–5 days.

- **Menopausal** women who are taking a cyclic estrogen, should have the goal to wean off of the synthetic hormone. Apply one pump per day for 25 days and then stop for 3 to 5 days. They should, at the same time, cut the amount of estrogen in half each month over three months. For example, the first month take the estrogen every other day; the second month take it every third day, and so on. *For women taking both estrogen and progestin, work in conjuction with a health-care professional to stop the progestin as soon as possible and take the estrogen and progesterone as instructed above.*

- One pump (20 mg.) is an average of what the body produces naturally. Some women need more than 20 mg. (or one pump daily) because of lifestyle, diet, or because their body would naturally produce more. If, after using one pump per day during the first month, you don't experience some relief from symptoms, try adding another pump. Use one pump in the morning and one at night. *Please note that it takes 3–6 cycles to experience the full benefits of bio-identical progesterone. You didn't get out of balance overnight, and you won't get back into balance overnight.*

- When you begin using bioidentical progesterone, you may experience **magnified symptoms** for a short while. Just know that this is your body's natural response and will subside as your hormones achieve balance.

- Some women may experience a little breakthrough bleeding. This is a signal that the body is using the progesterone cream to achieve balance.

- Ladies who are still having monthly periods should see their periods become more regular and PMS symptoms diminish as they use the cream. This can take 3–6 cycles.

- Listen to your body. During times of stress, you may need to increase your dose. Likewise, after 6–12 months, many women can decrease their dose to ½ pump per day.

- Remember to regularly rotate where you apply the cream. Use different sites such as the inside of the arms, the chest, neck, face, palms of the hands, and the soles of the feet. Make sure that the area is clean. *Never apply progesterone over a petroleum based cream.* (Look at the ingredients of the cream for the words mineral oil or petroleum base.) The hormone will not penetrate the petroleum layer **and** the petroleum will increase estrogen dominance.

- For women who are experiencing severe symptoms such as hot flashes and vaginal dryness, there is a bio-identical progesterone available which has additional natural herbs. The herbs act as phytoestrogens or natural plant estrogens which help women who are experiencing hot flashes or vaginal dryness. If you use the Phytoprolief (progesterone with additional herbs), you may begin to transition to the regular progesterone after the first 2–3 months of use if the hot flashes and vaginal dryness has subsided. If the symptoms have not diminished after a few months you may increase to two pumps a day if needed. You may also want to add some menopause formula supplements. *The desired goal is to wean off of the phytoestrogens (Phytorelief and menopause formula) and use the least amount of progesterone cream that will maintain your hormone balance.*

- For women who are not regularly having a period or no period at all (which would include ladies who have had a hysterectomy), then use progesterone for 25 days of the calendar month. Initially (one or two months), you may need to use one pump of the cream twice a day but one pump a day thereafter should be sufficient.

Endnotes

Chapter 3

[1]Loretta Walker, "Headaches, Hormones, and Other Hot Issues Over 40! (Part 1)," *Christian Womanhood*, April 2005, 11-12.

[2]Loretta Walker, "Headaches, Hormones, and Other Hot Issues Over 40! (Part 2)," *Christian Womanhood*, May 2005, 11-12.

Chapter 5

[1]Diana Schwarzbein, M.D., *The Schwarzbein Principle—The Program* (Deerfield Beach: Health Communications, Inc., 2004) 7.

Chapter 6

[1]Diana Schwarzbein, M.D., *The Schwarzbein Principle II—The Transition* (Deerfield Beach: Health Communications, Inc., 2002) 16, 17.

[2]*The Schwarzbein Principle—The Program*, 3.

Chapter 7

[1]http://www.vivo.colostate.edu/hbooks/path-phys/endocrine/basics/hormones.html

Chapter 8

[1]*The Schwarzbein Principle—The Program*, 13.

Chapter 10

[1]Lorraine Day, M.D., *Diseases Don't Just Happen!* (Thousand Palms: Rockford Press, 1998) Video.

Chapter 11

[1]*Diseases Don't Just Happen!*

[2]David L. Katz, M.D. "Does Sleep Affect Your Weight?" *Woman's World*, 29 August 2006, 17.

[3]*Diseases Don't Just Happen!*

Chapter 12

BBC Internet, http://www.bbc.co.uk.

Chapter 13

[1]Dr. John Lee. *What Your Doctor May Not Tell You about Premenopause* (New York: Time Warner Book Group, 2004) 46, 47.

[2]www.womensvibranthealth.libraryonhealth.com.

[3]*Ibid.*

Chapter 15

[1]Frieda Cowling, "The Missing Ingredient," *Christian Womanhood*, Vol. 30, No. 3, (June 2004), 17.

[2]Dr. Jack Schaap, *Opening the Door to the Unclean Spirits* (Hammond: Hyles Publications, 2005) 62.

Chapter 16

[1]Cindy Schaap, "Living on the Bright Side, Part II," *Christian Womanhood*, Vol. 30, No. 11, (March 2004), 9.

[2]*Opening the Door to the Unclean Spirits*, 53-54.
3 *Ibid.*, 84, 85.

Other Sources Consulted

Agaston, Arthur, M.D *The South Beach Diet* New York: St. Martin's Press, 2003.

Balch, James F., M.D. and Mark Stengler, N.D. *Prescription for Natural Cures* Hoboken: John Wiley Sons, Inc., 2004.

Balch, Phyllis A. CNC. *Prescription for Herbal Healing* New York: Penguin Putnam, Inc., 2002.

Calbom, Cherie, Maureen Keane. *Juicing for Life.* Honesdale: Paragon Press, 1992.

Cowling, Frieda. "The Missing Ingredient." *Christian Womanhood.* June 2004.

Day, Lorraine, M.D. *Diseases Don't Just Happen!* Video. Thousand Palms: Rockford Press, 1998.

Kordich, Jay. *The Juiceman's Power of Juicing.* New York: Warner Books, 1993.

Larson, David E., M.D. Editor-in-Chief. *Mayo Clinic Family Health Book*, New York: William Morrow and Company, Inc., 1990.

Lee, John R. M.D., with Virginia Hopkins. *What Your Doctor May Not Tell You About Menopause.* New York: Time Warner Book Group, 2004.

Lee, John R. M.D., Jesse Hanley, M.D., and Virginia Hopkins. *What Your Doctor May Not Tell You About Premenopause.* New York: Time Warner Book Group, 1999.

Malkmus, Dr. George H. *God's Way to Ultimate Health.* Shelby: Halleluja Acres Publishing, 1994.

Malkmus, Rhonda J. *Recipes for Life from God's Garden.* Shelby: Halleluja Acres Publishing, 1998.

McGraw, Dr. Phil. *The Ultimate Weight Solution The 7 Keys to Weight Loss Freedom.* New York: Free Press, 2003.

Nelson, Miriam E., Ph.D. with Sarah Wernick, Ph.D. *Strong Women Stay Slim* New York: Bantom, 1998.

Schaap, Cindy. "Living on the Bright Side, Part II." *Christian Womanhood*. March 2004.

Schwarzbein, Diana, M.D. *The Schwarzbein Principle—The Program*. Deerfield Beach: Health Communications, Inc., 2004.

Schwarzbein, Diana, M.D., with Marilyn Brown. *The Schwarzbein Principle II—The Transition*. Deerfield Beach: Health Communications, Inc., 2002.

Shames, Richard, M.D. and Karilee Shames, PhD, R.N. *Feeling Fat, Fuzzy, or Frazzled?* New York: Hudson Street Press, 2005.

Shoman, Mary J. *Living Well with Hypothyroidism*. New York: HarperCollins Publishers, Inc., 2000.

Somers, Suzanne. *Fast & Easy*. New York: Crown Publishing Group, 2002.

Trudeau, Kevin. *Natural Cures "They" Don't Want You to Know About*. Elk Grove Village: Alliance Publishing Group, Inc., 2004.

Wilson, James L., N.D., D.C., Ph.D. *Adrenal Fatigue The 21st Century Stress Syndrome*. Petaluma: Smart Publications, 2004.